Kennerley Bankes's
Clinical Ophthalmology

Kennerley Bankes's
Clinical
Ophthalmology

A Text and Colour Atlas

Fourth Edition

Edited by

G. G. W. Adams

Consultant Ophthalmic Surgeon
Moorfields Eye Hospital
London, UK

A. D. Hubbard

Specialist Registrar in Ophthalmology
South West Thames Region
London, UK

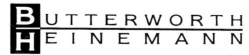

OXFORD   AUCKLAND   BOSTON   JOHANNESBURG   MELBOURNE   NEW DELHI

Butterworth-Heinemann
Linacre House, Jordan Hill, Oxford OX2 8DP
225 Wildwood Avenue, Woburn, MA 01801-2041
A division of Reed Educational and Professional Publishing Ltd

A member of the Reed Elsevier Group

First edition Longman Group 1982
Second edition Longman Group 1987
Third edition Longman Group 1994
Reprinted 1994
Fourth edition 1999

British Library Cataloguing in Publication Data
A catalogue record for this book is available from the British Library

Library of Congress Cataloguing in Publication Data
A catalogue record for this book is available from the Library of Congress

ISBN 0 7506 3908 3

Typeset by E & M Graphics, Midsomer Norton, Bath
Printed in Great Britain at the University Press, Cambridge

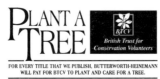

Contents

Preface to the Fourth Edition

This book aims to provide a current, concise, easily comprehensible guide to eye disease. Basic examination techniques are covered in detail and special attention is given to common conditions, such as red eye and cataract, and conditions requiring prompt recognition and urgent specialist referral.

Ophthalmological instrumentation and surgical techniques are described, and treatment regimens for conditions that require urgent intervention by the non-specialist.

The fourth edition of this book has a thoroughly updated text and many new illustrations. There are new chapters on ocular associations of systemic disease and paediatric problems as well as increased detail in several chapters, including description of refractive surgical techniques and a more comprehensive coverage of neuro-ophthalmology. An increased emphasis has been placed on the importance of ocular anatomy and physiology in understanding eye disorders.

It is hoped that this book will suit the needs of medical, orthoptic and optometry students as well as general practitioners, optometrists, casualty officers, ophthalmic nurses and those embarking on a career in ophthalmology.

London, 1999   G. G. W. A.
                                                A. D. H.

Preface to the First Edition

This book is written for those requiring some specialized knowledge of ophthalmology in their work and it is hoped that the needs of medical students, general practitioners and those beginning a career in ophthalmology will be met. Optometry students and optometrists have a need for a basic book in ophthalmology and it is hoped that this book will fulfil their requirements. There is much sophistication of instrumentation and surgery in ophthalmology which often obscures the fundamental unchanging facts and principles of the subject. All that is not essential for the non-specialist has been omitted, but conversely it is hoped that the vital fundamental information for clinical practice and reference is contained in this book. The book contains many colour illustrations, together with a few diagrams which assume a basic knowledge of anatomy and physiology. One chapter on rapid changes in refractive errors has the optometry student and optometrist much in mind, but may also prove of interest to the medical practitioner. Where appropriate, detailed treatments are given because the general medical practitioner often has to give the primary ophthalmological treatment.

London, 1982   J. L. K. B.

Acknowledgements

We are pleased and honoured to be asked by the family of the late Mr Kennerley Bankes and his publishers to undertake a new edition of his very successful textbook of clinical ophthalmology. We are extremely grateful for all the support and encouragement we have received in this project and would particularly like to thank Miss Cyrilla Chatfield, who has been associated with all editions, for her help in the preparation of the book.

We trust that this new update will maintain the high standards of previous editions.

1 Examination of the eye: use of instruments

A careful history and examination of a patient with an ophthalmic complaint will usually lead to a clear diagnosis being made without any special investigations being required. An understanding of the anatomy of the eye is helpful when dealing with ophthalmic conditions (Figs 1.1 and 1.2).

History

- Details should be taken of the site, duration, frequency and associated features of the complaint
- A past ophthalmic history should be obtained
- A past medical history, including that of medication and any allergies, should be noted
- Any family history of eye disease should be noted
- In children, a pre-birth and developmental history should be taken.

Examination

A careful **inspection of face and eyelids** will reveal any abnormalities or asymmetry.

ESTIMATION OF VISUAL ACUITY

The estimation of visual acuity in adults and older children is usually performed by using a Snellen chart, which consists of rows of letters diminishing in size from the top of the chart downward. Each row of letters is designated by a ratio of the test distance of 6 m (or 20 ft in North America) to the distance at which a normal person could read that size letter. Hence the top letter on the chart is designated 6/60 because a normal person could read that large letter at 60 m, and the

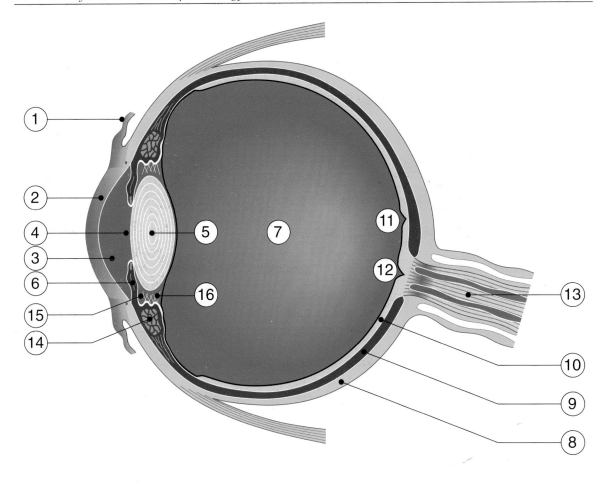

Horizontal section of the eye

1 Conjunctiva	9 Choroid
2 Cornea	10 Retina
3 Anterior chamber	11 Fovea (centralis)
4 Pupil	12 Optic disk
5 Lens	13 Optic nerve
6 Iris	14 Ciliary body
7 Vitreous body	15 Posterior chamber
8 Sclera	16 Zinn's zonule

Figure 1.1
Horizontal section of the eye.
(Reproduced with kind
permission of the Hoya
Corporation, Japan)

lowest line of letters on the chart is designated 6/6 (20/20 in
North America) which is the standard normal vision and the
size of letter seen by a normal person at 6 m. Some charts go
down as far as 6/5 or even 6/4 (Fig. 1.3).

The patient sits 6 m from the test chart or in smaller rooms
a 3-m reversing image with a mirror is used. Any necessary

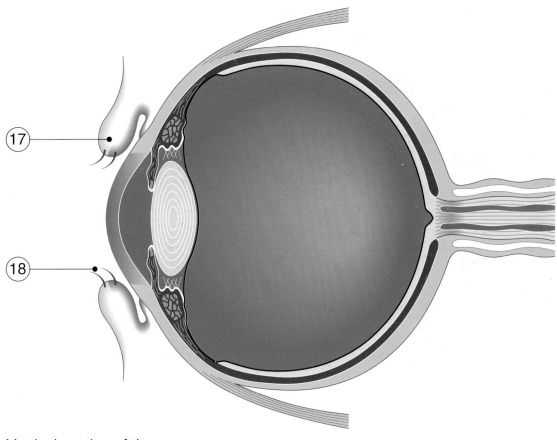

Vertical section of the eye

17 Eyelid
18 Eyelashes

Figure 1.2
Vertical section of the eye.
(Reproduced with kind
permission of the Hoya
Corporation, Japan)

distance spectacles should be worn for this essentially distance test. If glasses have been forgotten or if the acuity is reduced a pinhole test should be utilised. If even the top letter of the chart cannot be read then the patient should be brought closer to the chart and the vision re-checked. If the top letter is correctly identified at 3 m the acuity would be 3/60. If not seen at 3 m or closer the examiner should hold up a hand at 1 m and ask the patient to identify the number of fingers being displayed. A correct reply indicates count fingers (CF) vision. If the patient cannot count fingers a hand is moved in front of the eye and the patient is asked if any movement can be detected. This designates hand movement vision (HM). If

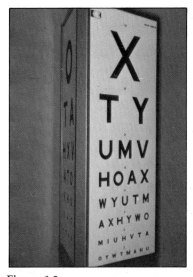

Figure 1.3
The Snellen chart

hand movements cannot be seen then it should be assessed whether or not the patient can see light (perception of light, PL or no perception of light, NPL). For illiterate patients and those unfamiliar with the Roman alphabet, letter Es of the standard test type facing in different directions may be used, with the patient indicating by hand the directions of the legs of the E. For young children aged 3 years and over the Sheridan–Gardiner test is excellent. The examiner holds at 6 m distance a card on which is a single test letter, and the child is asked to point to the matching letter on another card. The letter does not have to be named but merely matched with one on the child's own card (Fig. 1.4). This technique may also be used to match letters on a full Snellen chart. For children under 3 years picture recognition tests such as Kay cards may be useful. For smaller, preverbal children, preferential looking tests such as Keeler or Cardiff cards are very helpful. Preferential looking tests are based on children being more interested in patterned than in unpatterned targets so, if a child can see, the eyes or head will move towards the patterned rather than the plain card when both are presented simultaneously. Cards that are progressively more difficult to resolve are presented in order to assess the level of acuity.

Pinhole test

Looking through a tiny hole in a card held close to the eye is useful when testing visual acuity where a high refractive

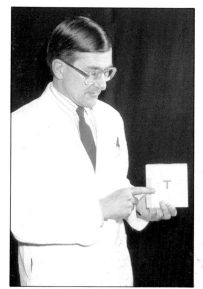

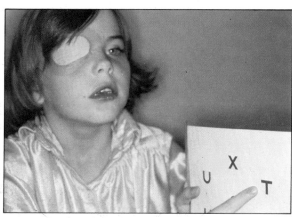

Figure 1.4
The Sheridan–Gardiner test

error is present and the patient's spectacles are not available. The hole in the card (easily made by pushing a pin through a card with a diameter of about 50 mm) allows only central light rays into the eye and eliminates the blurring of vision due to the refractive error. In general an improved visual acuity through a pinhole indicates that a refractive error, rather than a pathological condition, is the likely cause of the reduced visual acuity.

ANTERIOR SURFACE OF THE EYE

Inspection of the cornea and conjunctiva should be done with a good light or torch. The ophthalmologist uses a slit lamp microscope to obtain a magnified view (Fig. 1.5). If this is not available a magnifying loupe or a magnifying light, such as is found in many Accident and Emergency Departments, should be used (Fig. 1.6).

The **anterior chamber** of the eye can really only satisfactorily be examined in detail using a slit lamp although

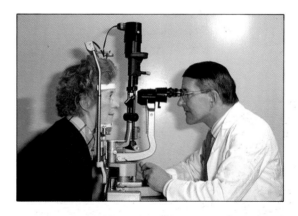

Figure 1.5
The slit lamp microscope

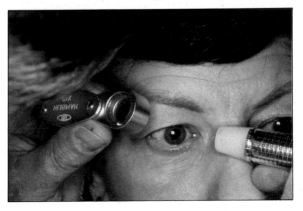

Figure 1.6
Examining the outer eye with a simple magnifier

examination with a torch will reveal any blood (hyphaema) or white cell (hypopyon) accumulation. With a slit lamp depth of the anterior chamber can be assessed, as can its activity, e.g. the presence of cells or flare as seen in iritis.

Intraocular pressure can only be measured by using specialist equipment such as an applanation tonometer attached to a slit lamp, or a pneumotonometer (air puff) used by many optometrists. In acute glaucoma with a high eye pressure, the eye may feel hard to the touch. Digital palpation, however, cannot be used to estimate more moderate elevations in eye pressure.

Pupils are normally round and equal in size. Any size or shape anomaly should be noted and the direct light, consensual light and convergence pupil reflexes tested. In eliciting the light pupil reflexes the light should be shone on the central retina (macula) and not obliquely. The convergence reflex is best determined by asking the patient to look at a particular point across the room and then look at a near object rapidly. A **relative afferent pupillary defect** is looked for by rapidly alternating the light source from one eye to the other. Normally both pupils should constrict in response to light; however in an eye with optic nerve or retinal damage the response is slower, and on swinging the light source from eye to eye the affected pupil will dilate when the light is brought back rapidly from the normal to the abnormal eye.

Ocular motility should be examined in all positions of gaze by asking the patient to follow a fixation target or pen torch to exclude any limitation of movement. Patients should be asked if they are aware of double vision in any position of gaze (Figs 1.7 and 1.8).

VISUAL FIELDS

Accurate plotting of visual fields by various static and kinetic perimetry machines is available to the specialist but a simple estimation of the field of vision can be obtained by the confrontation test. The patient and examiner are seated facing each other at the same level. The patient covers one eye with the palm of the hand and is asked to fix his or her gaze on the examiner's nose (a suitable fixation point). The examiner's opposite eye is similarly covered and from the periphery of

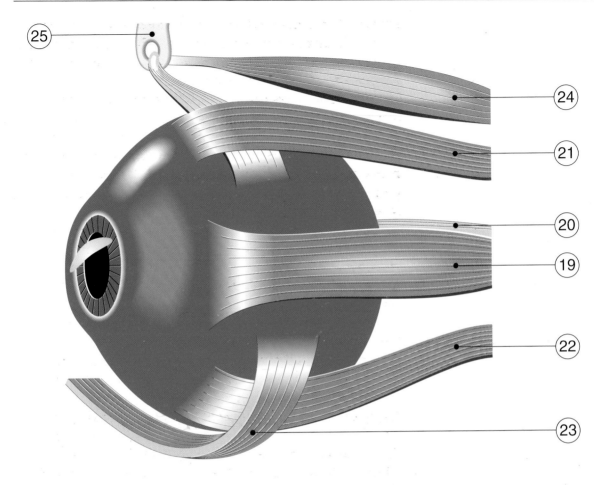

Extrinsic muscles of the eye

19	Lateral rectus	23	Inferior oblique
20	Medial rectus	24	Superior oblique
21	Superior rectus	25	Trochlea
22	Inferior rectus		

Figure 1.7
Extrinsic (extraocular) muscles of
the eye. (Reproduced with kind
permission of the Hoya
Corporation, Japan)

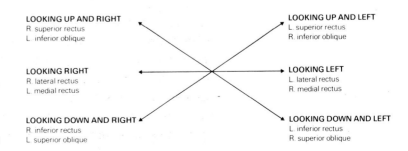

LOOKING UP AND RIGHT
R. superior rectus
L. inferior oblique

LOOKING UP AND LEFT
L. superior rectus
R. inferior oblique

LOOKING RIGHT
R. lateral rectus
L. medial rectus

LOOKING LEFT
L. lateral rectus
R. medial rectus

LOOKING DOWN AND RIGHT
R. inferior rectus
L. superior oblique

LOOKING DOWN AND LEFT
L. inferior rectus
R. superior oblique

Figure 1.8
The six cardinal positions of gaze

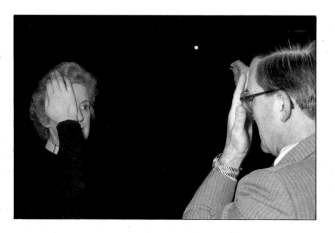

Figure 1.9
The confrontation field test

the visual field, each direction in turn, the examiner brings in a bright test-object which is a small white or red ball on a long pin (a hat pin). This test can be surprisingly accurate with practice, and is especially useful for a rapid field of vision screening when a central scotoma or hemianopia is suspected (Fig. 1.9).

FUNDUS EXAMINATION

The fundus of the eye is viewed using an ophthalmoscope (either direct or indirect) or alternatively by using a condensing lens with the patient seated at the slit lamp. With the conventional direct ophthalmoscope only one eye is used for observation which therefore does not allow a three-dimensional view. The binocular indirect ophthalmoscope is a specialist instrument that allows a stereoscopic or three-dimensional view of the interior of the eye. All forms of fundoscopy are easier after the pupil has been dilated and this is best achieved with tropicamide 1% eye drops which are short acting. In certain patients particularly diabetics who dilate poorly phenylephrine drops 2.5% may need to be used in addition. The patient should be warned not to drive for about 2 hours following pupil dilatation.

Ideally ophthalmoscopy should be carried out in a darkened room with the patient and examiner seated facing each other at the same level. The examiner's hand should be placed gently on the patient's forehead with the thumb over the patient's brow and upper eyelid. To examine the patient's right eye the examiner uses his or her own right eye and places the left hand on the patient's forehead. This is reversed

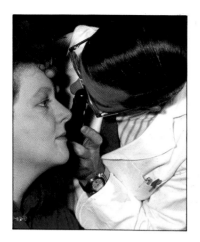

Figure 1.10
Using the direct ophthalmoscope

for examination of the left eye. The examiner's thumb over the brow and upper eyelid allows the eyelid to be elevated to avoid the eyelashes obstructing the view (Fig. 1.10).

With the patient's gaze fixed on a point across the room the ophthalmoscope light is shone into the pupil and a red fundus reflection or reflex will be observed. With a +5 or +6 lens in the ophthalmoscope rack held at about 120 mm from the eye any opacities in the cornea, lens and vitreous will be visible as silhouettes against the red fundus reflex. This is particularly useful in detecting cataract. The ophthalmoscope is then brought slowly closer to the patient's eye (15 mm is satisfactory) and the ophthalmoscope lens is adjusted to approximately zero until the fundus comes into view. Adjustments to the rack of lenses on the ophthalmoscope will be required to obtain a clear fundus picture depending on the refractive error of the patient and the examiner. The optic disc should first be inspected, then the macula, the retinal vessels and finally each quadrant of the fundus in turn. Ophthalmoscopy requires constant practice.

Difficulties in visualising the fundus can occur when:

- The ophthalmoscope light is poor
- The pupil is too small
- There is too much light scatter from the corneal surface
- The room is inadequately darkened
- High myopia is present; this causes the view with the direct opthalmoscope to be more highly magnified leading to difficulties with orientation. This can be overcome by performing ophthalmoscopy with patients wearing their distance spectacles
- There are opacities in the media, especially cataract, which obscure a good fundus view.

2

Refractive problems

Anatomy

Parallel light rays impinging upon the eye need to be brought to a point of focus on the retina in order to be perceived as a clear image. This process involves the bending or **refraction** of light rays as they pass though the eye. The majority of this refraction is performed by the cornea with the lens being responsible for a lesser degree. The lens is held in position by fine suspensory zonule fibres which arise from the ciliary body and attach into the basement membrane capsule surrounding the lens. Changes in tension exerted by the zonule fibres, caused by contraction or relaxation of the ciliary muscle, allow the lens to alter its surface curvature and thickness to focus images clearly on the retina.

Refractive errors

If the eye does not accurately focus light rays onto the retina at the back of the eye then there is a refractive error. If images are focused sharply on the retina this is called emmetropia or normal sight. Approximately 50 per cent of the population suffer from reduced unaided acuity and require the use of corrective lenses. The **dioptre** (reciprocal of the focal length of the eye) is the unit of lens power used for spectacle correction.

Hypermetropia or **long sight** is where the eye is too short and light is focused behind the retina. Most children are born hypermetropic but become less so with age and this eventually leads to emmetropia in the majority of cases. Most children and young adults can overcome a small hypermetropic error by increasing the power of the crystalline lens (**accommodation**; see Chapter 4). As the power of accommodation is lost with age, such patients usually require distance glasses in middle adult life. Hypermetropia is corrected with convex or positive lenses (Fig. 2.1).

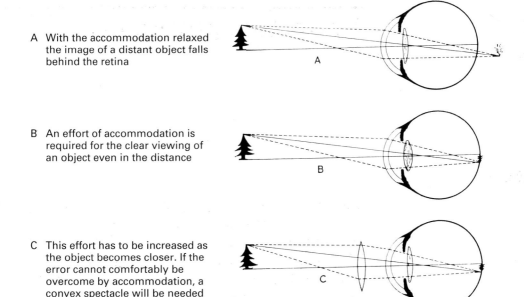

A   With the accommodation relaxed the image of a distant object falls behind the retina

B   An effort of accommodation is required for the clear viewing of an object even in the distance

C   This effort has to be increased as the object becomes closer. If the error cannot comfortably be overcome by accommodation, a convex spectacle will be needed

Figure 2.1 Hypermetropia

Presbyopia is an age-related variant of hypermetropia. It is caused by loss of elasticity of the crystalline lens which reduces its power of accommodation. This results in near objects being out of focus and a requirement for reading spectacles.

Myopia or **short sight** is where the eye is too long and light is focused in front of the retina. Distance objects are blurred but near objects can be seen clearly. Myopia occurs in approximately one in five adults, often starts in adolescence and usually stabilises in the twenties. Myopia is corrected with concave or negative lenses (Fig. 2.2).

Astigmatism is where the eye does not focus light evenly usually due to the cornea of the eye being more curved in one direction than another. The eye is sometimes described as resembling a rugby ball rather than a football when explaining the condition to patients. It may occur on its own or be associated with myopia or hypermetropia. Astigmatism is corrected with cylindrical lenses.

Refractive errors if corrected can improve visual acuity. Low errors of refraction may not require treatment but if acuity is reduced correction will improve vision. A refractive error is often termed 'high' (i.e. high myopia, high hypermetropia) if the correcting spectacle lens is ≥ ±6 dioptres.

A The image of a distant object falls in front of the retina and any effort of accommodation will only increase the blurring

B Near objects, on the other hand, are seen clearly with little or no accommodation

C For clear distant sight a concave spectacle is needed

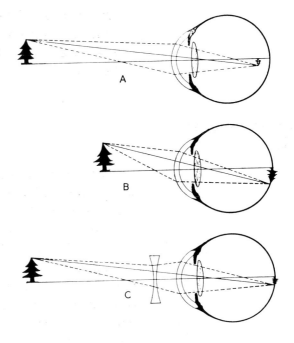

Figure 2.2 Myopia

Certain ocular conditions are related to refractive error, with retinal detachment being more common in high myopia and acute glaucoma in high hypermetropia. **Anisometropia** is present when there is a difference in refractive error between the two eyes.

Refractive errors can be corrected with:

1. **Glasses.** Many patients dislike glasses because they are uncomfortable to wear or may be inconvenient in certain occupational or sporting settings. Children may be sensitive about wearing spectacles. Plastic spectacle lenses should always be prescribed for children because of the risk of ocular damage if glass lenses are shattered.

2. **Contact lenses.** These can be soft (daily wear or extended wear), semi-rigid gas permeable, or hard. There is a significant risk of ocular infection with extended wear soft contact lenses. Patients should be thoroughly instructed in handling and cleaning techniques. If a contact lens-wearing patient develops a red eye the lens should be removed and glasses used instead. Many of these problems will be contact lens-related and will settle after removing the lens. If the eye does not settle spon-

taneously specialist advice should be sought. All patients who use contact lenses should have a back-up pair of spectacles.
3. Surgery.

Refractive surgical techniques

Corneal microsurgical techniques are mainly used to treat myopia and astigmatism. Treatment for hypermetropia is less well developed. The procedures work by altering the anterior surface of the cornea; by flattening it in patients with myopia, increasing the curvature in cases of hypermetropia, and by flattening only certain areas in cases of astigmatism. The aim is to improve the unaided distance acuity. Patients can be considered for refractive surgery if they are over 21 years with a stable refraction in glasses or contact lenses for correction of distance vision. They should be free of any other significant eye disease and be in good general health.

The most commonly used refractive surgical techniques are:

- **Radial keratotomy (RK)**. In RK a series of incisions to 95 per cent of its depth are made in the anterior cornea in a spoke-like fashion. This flattens the central cornea thereby reducing myopia. The main problems are fluctuating vision and a weakened cornea.
- **Astigmatic keratotomy**. Surgical incisions are made in different configurations in the corneal periphery to treat astigmatism.
- **Automated lamellar keratoplasty (ALK)**. In ALK two incisions are made with a microkeratome. The first cuts a corneal flap and the second removes a layer of underlying cornea before the corneal flap is repositioned. The consequent reduction in corneal curvature reduces myopia.
- **Photorefractive keratectomy (excimer laser, PRK)**. The ultraviolet excimer laser is used to reshape the anterior surface of the cornea over the pupil area whilst retaining its strength and structure. It is used to treat low to moderate myopia and astigmatism. At the present time treatment for hypermetropia is in its infancy. Complications of excimer

laser include the following:

- Discomfort or pain after the surgery
- Light sensitivity and haloes
- Corneal scarring particularly after treatment of higher amounts of myopia; this may lead to problems with night vision and loss of best corrected visual acuity
- Over/under-correction.

- **Laser-assisted in situ keratomileusis (LASIK)**. LASIK is one of the newest refractive procedures. It is considered most effective for patients with higher levels of refractive error and is said to produce less risk of corneal scarring and more predictable results. In this technique a corneal flap is lifted by microkeratome, excimer laser is applied to the underlying cornea, and the flap is then replaced.
- **Other surgical techniques**. Less common techniques for treating high levels of myopia are clear lens extraction and insertion of a contact lens on to the surface of the crystalline lens.

Rapid changes in refractive error

When a refractive error changes over a short period such as days or weeks then an underlying cause should always be sought. Refractive errors usually vary only slowly over the years except in growing children. Causes for consideration include the following:

- **Senile cataract**. Rapidly advancing myopia may occur due to an increasing refractive index of the lens.
- **Diabetes mellitus**. Fluctuation in blood sugar, and hence aqueous sugar level, may cause a change in the refractive index of the lens. An undiagnosed diabetic may become rapidly myopic over a few weeks because of the increased blood sugar level. A rapid fall in blood sugar level with treatment will cause hypermetropia and a consequent blurring of near vision. Sometimes a newly treated diabetic will complain of increased reading difficulty having been accustomed to the comfortable near vision of myopia due to an increased blood sugar level. Because of these rapid changes in refractive error newly treated or unstable

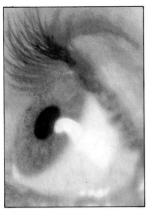

(a)

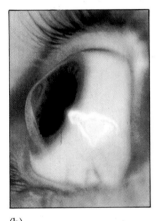

(b)

Figure 2.3
(a) Normal eye
(b) Keratoconus

diabetics should either wait for spectacles or be given temporary ones until the diabetes has been stabilised.

- **Keratoconus**. The onset of keratoconus (conical cornea) may be rapid and an increase in myopia and astigmatism over a period of weeks is characteristic. Keratoconus should always be considered where there is rapid variation in astigmatism particularly in adolescence and in early adulthood (Figs 2.3 a and b).

- **Subluxation of the lens**. A change in the position of the crystalline lens due to subluxation can induce a rapid change in refractive error and consequent blurred vision. In a simple subluxation, when the lens is constantly moving, a change in the refractive error may occur every few minutes, being hypermetropic as the lens moves backwards and myopic as the lens moves forwards (see Chapter 9). An iris or ciliary body neoplasm may also cause displacement of the lens giving similar changes in refractive error.

- **Eye drops**. Most eye drops will have been prescribed for ophthalmic treatment. Occasionally they get used mistakenly by other people or very rarely drops for nasal use can inadvertently be instilled into the eye. Spasm of accommodation caused by pilocarpine induces an artificial myopia. Patients on miotic drops should only be prescribed spectacles when they are on a regular and stable treatment regimen. Relaxation of accommodation with the use of cycloplegic or mydriatic eye drops will be accompanied by pupil dilatation and will induce a state of increased hypermetropia and blurring of near vision.

- **Eyelid lump**. External pressure on the eye from an eyelid swelling can induce astigmatism because of a slight distortion of the cornea.

3

Colour vision defects

Introduction

The retinal photoreceptor layer comprises two major class of cells termed **rods** and **cones**. Colour vision in humans is based on the presence of three classes of cone; red, green and blue. A person is trichromatic if all three systems are present, dichromatic if one system is absent and monochromatic if two are absent. A partial red defect is protonomaly, a green one is deuteranomaly, and a blue one a tritanomaly. If the system is completely absent these become protanopia, deuteranopia and tritanopia. Defective colour vision can be congenital or acquired.

CONGENITAL COLOUR VISION DEFECTS

In Western populations 8% of males and 0.5% of females have a defect of the red/green system inherited as an X-linked recessive trait. Achromotopsia or rod monochromatism is a stationary retinal disorder in which there is absence of all functional cones. It is associated with extremely poor vision, poor colour vision, photophobia and nystagmus.

ACQUIRED COLOUR VISION DEFECTS

Acquired colour vision defects can occur with advancing cataract, optic nerve disease or retinal disorders such as macular degeneration, toxic amblyopia, chronic glaucoma and diabetic retinopathy. Red/green abnormalities are usually associated with optic nerve problems and blue/yellow defects with macular disease and glaucoma.

Importance of colour deficiency

Colour deficiency cannot be treated, but it is important that it is recognised. It may have occupational implications because some jobs demand normal colour vision, for example civil and military pilots and those who work in shipping and on the railways.

Tests for colour vision defects

- **Isochromatic charts**. These charts consist of a number or letter made up of coloured dots on a background of differently coloured dots of equal brightness. The patient is required to identify the number or letter on the chart. The best known of these is the Ishihara test for red/green but

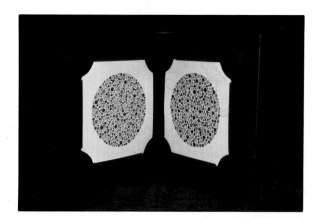

Figure 3.1
The Ishihara test

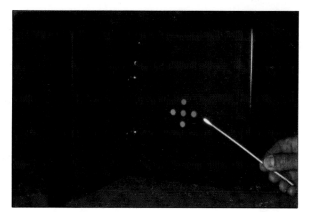

Figure 3.2
The City University Colour Vision Test

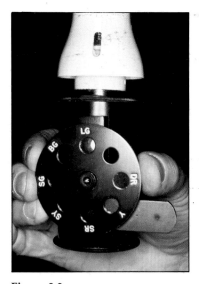

Figure 3.3
The Giles–Archer lantern test

other similar tests are the City University Colour Vision Test and the H-R-R test (Figs 3.1 and 3.2).

- *Lantern tests.* A number of lantern tests are in use in the aviation and transport industries. One simple and portable version is the Giles–Archer lantern test. The patient is asked to identify a succession of coloured lights used in the transport industries as signal lights (red, green, blue-green, yellow) (Fig. 3.3).

- **Formal electrodiagnostic colour contrast sensitivity tests**. These can be performed in specialist departments.

4

Age changes in the eye

A number of physiological changes occur in the eyes with increasing age. They are all harmless but should be recognised in order to distinguish them from pathological conditions.

Ageing of function

ACCOMMODATION

Accommodation is the increase in effectivity or power of the crystalline lens caused by contraction of the ciliary muscle. The ciliary muscle is innervated by the parasympathetic fibres of the third cranial nerve and its contraction causes a reduction in the tension on the lens zonule fibres, thus allowing the elastic lens to assume a more spherical (and powerful) shape. This process allows near objects to be focused on the retina.

Loss of elasticity of the lens with age leads to a gradual decline in accommodation and the condition known as **presbyopia**. Presbyopia usually becomes evident in middle adult life and causes blurring of vision for close objects. It is overcome by the wearing of near vision spectacles for reading, sewing, and other close work. Presbyopia has less effect on the myopic patient who is often able to continue to read without glasses throughout life.

DARK ADAPTATION

The ability of the retina to adapt to low levels of illumination occurs as a result of rhodopsin synthesis in the rod cells of the retina. Old people adapt at a slower rate to dark conditions (dark adaptation) and hence feel less secure in any darkened room or at night.

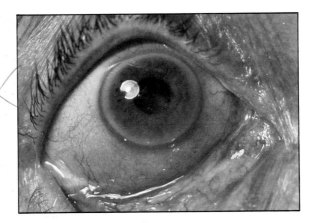

Figure 4.1
Arcus senilis of the cornea

Ageing of structure

ARCUS SENILIS OF THE CORNEA

The arcus senilis appears as a whitish ring in the periphery of the cornea with a clear zone separating it from the limbus. The appearance is due to deposition of phospholipids in the corneal periphery and can be seen in many people after late middle age. It is harmless and does not affect vision (Fig. 4.1). An arcus appearing in a younger patient may be associated with hyperlipidaemia.

PINGUECULA OF THE CONJUNCTIVA

Yellowish nodules on the nasal and temporal conjunctiva are frequently seen after middle age and consist of hyaline and lipid degenerative patches on the exposed part of the conjunctiva (Fig. 4.2). Pingueculae are harmless but may be considered a cosmetic blemish by some people, in which case they can be surgically removed.

VITREOUS

The vitreous humour is a clear, gel-like substance that fills the posterior four-fifths of the eye (vitreous cavity). Anteriorly it is apposed to the lens and peripherally and posteriorly to the retina. With age the vitreous becomes more liquid and the fine vitreous fibrils may come closer together giving rise to the

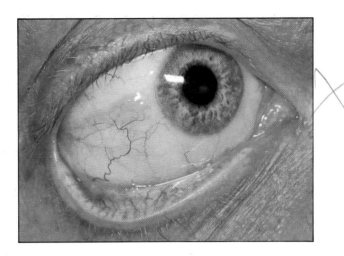

Figure 4.2
Pinguecula

appearance of condensations. These fibrillar condensations cause the symptom of floating hair-like opacities and the larger ones may be seen with the ophthalmoscope.

In middle life particularly the condition of **posterior vitreous detachment (PVD)** may occur. This gives rise to symptoms similar to retinal detachment; sudden onset of floating opacities, blurred vision and flashing lights (photopsia). PVD is a normal age-related degeneration where the vitreous becomes detached from the retina. The remaining collapsed vitreous is suspended within the vitreous cavity where it may be visualised by the patient as a 'floater'. As a PVD develops it may tug on the retina, causing the patient to experience flashing lights. As the vitreous detaches from the retina it occasionally causes a retinal tear which may subsequently lead to retinal detachment. The vitreous tends to degenerate at an earlier age in myopic patients.

Patients with symptoms of floaters and flashes require careful examination through a dilated pupil to distinguish between a retinal detachment or tear which requires immediate treatment, and a posterior vitreous detachment which requires no treatment except for explanation and reassurance. The symptoms of posterior vitreous detachment usually resolve after several weeks or months. The light flashes, or photopsia, resolve when there is separation of the vitreous from the areas of retinal adhesion and the vitreous therefore ceases to tug the peripheral retina. Vitreous opacities may persist indefinitely but gradually the patient learns to ignore them.

FUNDUS

With increasing age, arteriosclerosis of the retinal vessels occurs. This may be observed in the fundus as narrowing of the retinal arterioles and occasional variations in calibre.

EYELIDS

Decrease in elastic tissue of the skin and loss of muscle tone will produce the typical appearance of age, namely loose skin folds of the eyelids or 'baggy' eyelids (blepharochalasis) with skin wrinkling. For cosmetic reasons these loose skin folds may occasionally be surgically removed.

5 Eyelid conditions

Anatomy and physiology

The eyelids are modified mobile folds of skin with a firm tarsal plate of fibrous tissue in each to give strength and rigidity. Skin covers the outer part of the eyelid under which lies the orbicularis oculi muscle fibres supplied by the facial nerve (VIIth cranial nerve). Contraction of these fibres causes closure of the eyelids. Within each tarsal plate is a row of some 20 meibomian glands secreting an oily sebum from openings on the eyelid margin to form an oily layer over the tear film. The inner surface of the eyelids is lined with conjunctiva (tarsal conjunctiva), a mucous membrane, continuous with the conjunctiva on the anterior portion of the sclera (bulbar conjunctiva). Inserted into the upper portion of the tarsal plate is the levator palpebrae superioris muscle supplied by the oculomotor nerve (IIIrd cranial nerve). The levator muscle is responsible for raising the upper eyelid when the eye is open. The eyelids and the bony orbits provide vital protection for the eyes from external injury (Figs 5.1 and 5.2).

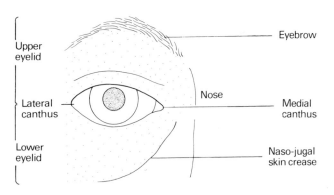

Figure 5.1
Surface markings of the eyelids

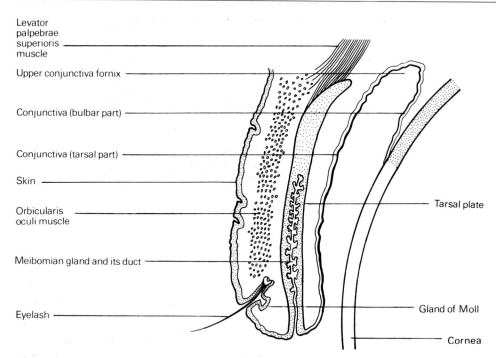

Levator palpebrae superioris muscle

Upper conjunctiva fornix

Conjunctiva (bulbar part)

Conjunctiva (tarsal part)

Skin

Orbicularis oculi muscle

Meibomian gland and its duct

Eyelash

Tarsal plate

Gland of Moll

Cornea

Figure 5.2
Vertical section through the eyelid

Eyelid conditions will be discussed under the following headings:

- Inflammatory eyelid conditions
- Degenerative and malpositioning eyelid conditions
- Eyelid tumours.

Inflammatory eyelid conditions

MEIBOMIAN CYST (OR CHALAZION)

This is a painless lump that can be felt in the eyelid, increasing in size over several days or weeks to about the size of a pea. The lump has mobile skin overlying it and consists of a collection of granulation tissue, probably as a result of trapped sebum secretion from the Meibomian glands in the eyelid (Fig. 5.3). If there is acute infection of a blocked Meibomian gland the lid swelling will be hot and tender and may discharge (infected Meibomian cyst). Following resolution of the infective episode a chalazion may remain.

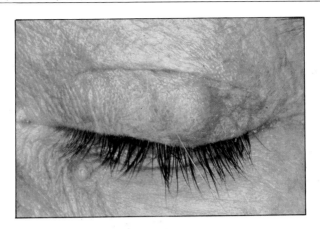

Figure 5.3
Meibomian cyst (chalazion)

Treatment

An infected Meibomian cyst is treated with topical or, occasionally oral antibiotics along with 'hot spoon bathing' (see below) to encourage the cyst to discharge. A very large infected cyst may require surgical incision. Some chalazions may resolve spontaneously over several weeks but the majority require incision and curettage removal.

STYE

A stye is an acute staphylococcal infection of the eyelash follicle presenting as a rapidly developing tender, red, discharging lump on the eyelid margin. It is identical to a small boil or skin furuncle (Fig. 5.4). With recurrent styes a blood sugar or urine test for diabetes mellitus should be carried out.

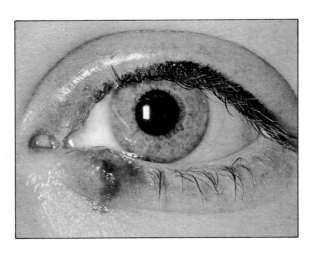

Figure 5.4
Stye

Treatment

Pulling the eyelash from the stye aids drainage of the pus and topical antibiotics are usually applied to the eye. A hot compress applied to the stye (by wrapping lint or cotton wool round the handle of a wooden spoon and wetting the cotton wool in hot water; 'hot spoon bathing') or steaming the face over a bowl of hot water relieves pain and allows the stye to discharge.

BLEPHARITIS

This is a chronic inflammation of the eyelid margins causing a bilateral redness, crusting and soreness of the eyelids. Most common in the younger age group it can however persist throughout life, waxing and waning in severity and eventually leading to loss of the eyelashes (Fig. 5.5). In most cases it is caused by staphylococcal infection, and it may be associated with acne rosacea.

Treatment

Lid toilet to remove the crusts and debris from the eyelids should be performed twice a day using a cotton bud and plain boiled water. If the lid margins are very greasy the addition of a drop of baby shampoo to the cleaning water may be helpful.

Topical antibiotic ointment applied to the eyelid margins twice a day after lid cleaning is useful when exacerbations occur. In particularly troublesome cases long-term low-dose oral antibiotics such as erythromycin or one of the

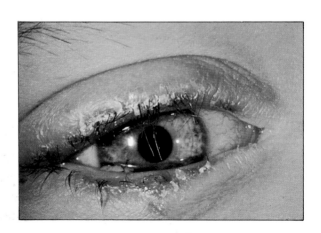

Figure 5.5
Blepharitis

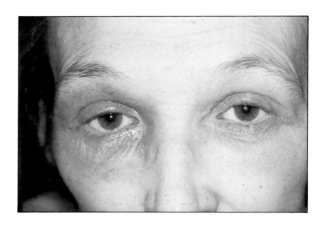

Figure 5.6
Allergic blepharitis

tetracyclines is helpful (250 mg b.d. for 6 weeks to 6 months may be necessary).

ALLERGIC BLEPHARITIS

Allergic blepharitis has a rapid onset over several hours with swelling of the lids and intense itching. It may occur in response to known allergies such as pollens, dust and eating shellfish or to makeup or eye drops. In the case of a contact allergy the swelling is usually confined to the area of contact with the skin (Fig. 5.6).

Treatment

Symptoms usually settle when there is no longer exposure to the causative allergen. Cold compresses to relieve the itching and swelling and topical or oral antihistamines may be useful.

Degenerative and malpositioning eyelid conditions

CYST OF MOLL

The Glands of Moll are very small sweat glands lying close to the eyelid margins. They form cystic swellings of the eyelids when obstructed. These cysts are initially small and translucent but enlarge over many months (Fig. 5.7).

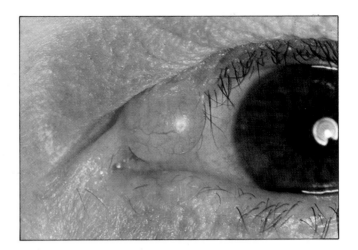

Figure 5.7
Cyst of Moll

Treatment

This consists of excising the cyst for cosmetic reasons or because of discomfort.

XANTHELASMA

Yellow lipid deposits in the skin of the eyelids are called xanthelasma. These yellow, soft, flat areas commence mainly on the nasal aspects of the eyelids and gradually increase in size over several years (Fig. 5.8). They are often associated with hyperlipidaemia, hence patients presenting with this condition should be assessed for an underlying cause.

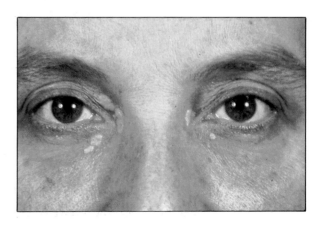

Figure 5.8
Xanthelasma of the eyelids

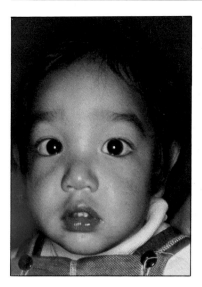

Figure 5.9
Epicanthus

Treatment

Simple excision of the xanthelasma under local anaesthetic produces a good cosmetic result but recurrences may occur especially where there is an underlying systemic cause.

EPICANTHUS

Many babies are born with an additional fold of skin called an epicanthus which extends from the nasal aspect of the upper eyelid to the lower eyelid at the medial canthus. It usually gradually disappears during the first 2 years of life with growth of the face (Fig. 5.9). In Oriental races it is a normal and recognised facial feature and persists throughout life.

The importance of recognising epicanthus lies in the fact that it can frequently give the impression of a convergent squint and careful examination to exclude the presence of a squint must be undertaken.

Treatment

Only when severe epicanthus persists into late infancy, especially when accompanied by congenital ptosis, is cosmetic surgery indicated. This may be performed at any time in childhood or early adult life.

ENTROPION

Senile involutional entropion is a common condition in elderly people. The lower eyelid turns inwards causing the eyelashes to abrade the cornea and conjunctiva. This gives rise to a painful, red and discharging eye (Fig. 5.10).

Entropion may less commonly occur secondary to scarring of the tarsal conjunctiva (cicatrical entropion), from ocular irritation from a foreign body or keratitis (spastic entropion) because of spasm of the orbicularis oculi muscle.

Treatment

Surgical repair is the only permanent cure for this condition, and is performed as an out-patient under local anaesthetic. To relieve the patient's symptoms whilst awaiting operation the skin of the lower eyelid may be pulled down and strapped onto the cheek with narrow tape each day.

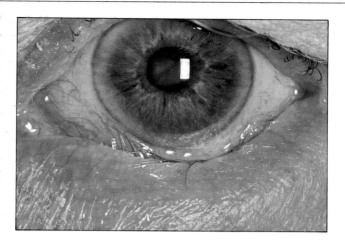

Figure 5.10
Entropion

ECTROPION

This is the opposite of entropion; the lower eyelid sags downwards and turns out leaving exposed tarsal conjunctiva. The appearance is that of a reddened, exposed tarsal conjunctiva with watering of the eye because the lower punctum is no longer apposed to the eye (Fig. 5.11).

Most ectropion occurs in elderly patients secondary to involutional changes in eyelid structure. Occasionally it may also occur as a result of scarring of the eyelid skin from chemical or thermal burns, chronic eczema, or as a result of paralysis of the facial nerve (VIIth cranial nerve).

Treatment

Symptomatic senile ectropion is treated by surgical repair of the lower eyelid performed under local anaesthetic as an out-patient.

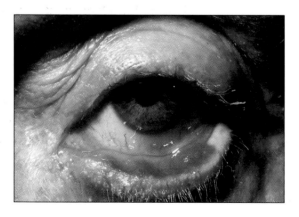

Figure 5.11
Ectropion

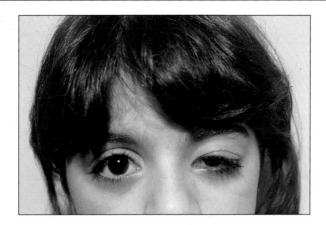

Figure 5.12
Ptosis

PTOSIS

This is drooping of the upper eyelid and may be congenital or acquired (Fig. 5.12). Congenital causes of ptosis are dealt with in Chapter 14. Acquired ptosis may be:

- **Involutional**. Age-related tissue laxity or disinsertion of the levator muscle complex is a common cause of senile ptosis
- **Neurogenic**. IIIrd nerve palsy or Horner's syndrome will cause ptosis often in association with other eye signs (see Chapters 13 and 12 respectively)
- **Myogenic**. Certain muscle disorders (e.g. dystrophia myotonica, ocular myopathy) may cause a ptosis often in association with poor eye closure and abnormalities of eye movement
- **Myasthenic**. Typically causes a fatiguable ptosis which worsens towards the end of the day (see Chapter 12)
- **Mechanical**. An eyelid swelling may cause a mechanical ptosis
- **Traumatic**. Damage to the levator muscle complex may result in ptosis.

Treatment

Various surgical approaches are available to correct a ptosis that is cosmetically unacceptable or interfering with vision. In certain patients 'ptosis props' attached to spectacles may be useful.

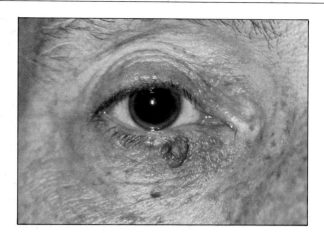

Figure 5.13
Papilloma of the eyelid

Eyelid tumours

PAPILLOMA

Simple squamous papillomas are common on the eyelid, as elsewhere on the skin, and may be single or multiple. They are skin-coloured lumps of varying size and may increase in size very slowly or remain unchanged for many years (Fig. 5.13).

Treatment

This consists of simple excision of the papilloma either for cosmetic reasons or to relieve discomfort of the eyelid.

BASAL CELL CARCINOMA (RODENT ULCER)

The rodent ulcer, deriving its name from the gradual 'gnawing away' of the skin, is the most common malignant tumour of the eyelids. It commences as a small lump anywhere on the eyelid and gradually increases in size over several months until it has an ulcerated centre bordered by a raised whitish edge. The rodent ulcer is prone to bleed easily and scab over the central portion. It steadily enlarges, eroding the skin and even the underlying bone as it does so. Any small lump on the skin that progressively enlarges and is prone to bleeding must be regarded as a likely rodent ulcer (Fig. 5.14).

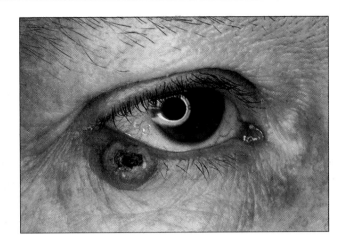

Figure 5.14
Basal cell carcinoma (rodent ulcer) of the eyelid

Treatment

Excision of the suspected rodent ulcer should be undertaken with a wide margin of normal skin being removed round the lump. Following the excision of a lid lesion reconstructive plastic surgery is required to restore the integrity of the lids which are essential in maintaining a healthy ocular surface. Radiotherapy is also an effective treatment but biopsy of the lump should be undertaken beforehand to establish the diagnosis.

SQUAMOUS CELL CARCINOMA

This is less common on the eyelids than basal cell carcinoma. An irregular, progressively enlarging lump, often at a

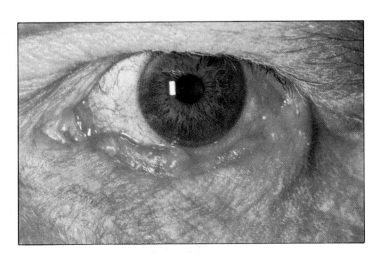

Figure 5.15
Squamous cell carcinoma of the eyelid

canthus, is the usual course of a squamous cell carcinoma. The lump often ulcerates and exudes fluid (Fig. 5.15). Lymph node enlargement from lymphatic spread is frequent (pre-auricular and submandibular nodes) and should be carefully looked for with any eyelid lump suspected of being malignant.

Treatment

Wide excision of the lump should be undertaken and where there is extensive eyelid involvement, major reconstructive plastic surgery may be required. Irradiation may also be necessary either on its own or in conjunction with surgery.

A note of caution should be sounded here. In the early stages squamous cell carcinoma (of the eyelid margins in particular) and basal cell carcinoma may appear as a single reddened area and be mistaken for blepharitis. However blepharitis is always a bilateral chronic condition, whereas carcinoma is unilateral, has a short history and is confined to one eyelid or canthus.

6

The lacrimal system

Anatomy and physiology

The lacrimal gland lies in the upper, outer quadrant of the orbit, protected by the bony orbital wall in its own fossa. Ducts from the lacrimal gland open in the upper conjunctival fornix and secrete tear fluid over the surface of the eye aided by the 'smearing' action of blinking. From the surface of the eye the tears leave by evaporation and via drainage into the lacrimal puncta, which are situated on the upper and lower eyelid margins about one quarter of the eyelid's length from the inner canthus. The puncta are two very small openings that drain tears into two corresponding canaliculi that run towards the nose just beneath the skin of the eyelids. The canaliculi join a dilated portion of the lacrimal passageway

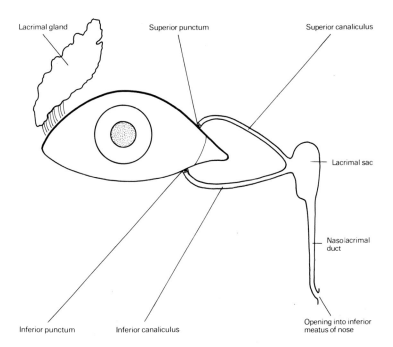

Lacrimal gland

Superior punctum

Superior canaliculus

Lacrimal sac

Nasolacrimal duct

Inferior punctum

Inferior canaliculus

Opening into inferior meatus of nose

Figure 6.1
Lacrimal passages

called the lacrimal sac which lies against the bone between the orbit and the nose. The nasolacrimal duct completes the passageway for tear fluid and runs downwards and backwards in the bone into the inferior meatus of the nose (Fig. 6.1). During blinking closure of the eyes by the orbicularis oculi muscle causes tears to be sucked from the eye into the lacrimal sac (lacrimal pump). When the eyes open the contents of the lacrimal sac pass down the nasolacrimal duct via gravity.

The following conditions of the lacrimal apparatus will be considered:

- Dry eyes
- Watery eyes
- Lacrimal gland disorders.

Dry eyes

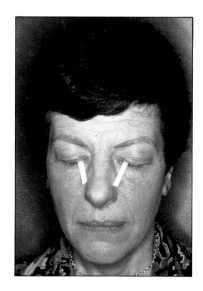

Figure 6.2
Schirmer's tear flow test

An abnormality of the tear film is one of the most common causes of chronic ocular irritation. Symptoms are caused by corneal drying and are usually mild burning and grittiness with normal vision. In severe tear deficiency however, symptoms can be very marked and poor vision or blindness may occur secondary to corneal damage.

Signs include a reduced tear meniscus on the lower eyelid margin, mucous threads, a lack-lustre cornea, fluorescein and rose bengal staining of the inferior cornea and conjunctiva, and reduced wetting on Schirmer's test. Schirmer's test entails placing standard filter paper strips in the lower conjunctival fornix and measuring the amount of wetting after 5 minutes. Less than 10 mm of wetting is abnormal (Fig. 6.2).

The normal tear film consists of an inner mucous layer derived from conjunctival goblet cells, an aqueous layer derived from the lacrimal gland (containing the antibacterial agent lyzozyme) and an outer lipid layer derived from the Meibomian glands of the eyelids. Abnormalities of any of these components may cause dry eye.

LACRIMAL GLAND DISEASE

Keratoconjunctivitis sicca arises due to a deficiency in aqueous tear production by the lacrimal gland. The cause is often due to senile atrophy of the lacrimal gland but may occur secondary to infiltration or inflammation of the lacrimal gland in sarcoidosis or connective tissue disease (especially rheumatoid arthritis; see Chapter 15). Certain drugs, including phenothiazines, antihistamines, anticholinergics and beta-blockers may cause dry eye by inducing lacrimal gland hyposecretion.

CONJUNCTIVAL SCARRING

Diseases such as Stevens–Johnson syndrome, ocular cicatritial pemphigoid and trachoma (see Chapter 15) often produce severe dry eyes secondary to conjunctival scarring which may obliterate lacrimal ductules in the upper conjunctival fornix and/or reduce mucus production by conjunctival goblet cells.

BLEPHARITIS

Blepharitis is frequently associated with dry eyes due to a combination of chronic infection and Meibomian gland dysfunction which interferes with tear film stability.

Treatment

If an underlying cause can be identified and treated dry eyes will often improve. First-line treatment is with artificial tear drops (such as Hypromellose) which may need to be instilled as often as once or twice hourly with severe symptoms. Gels (such as Viscotears) increase the contact time and therefore allow for less frequent application but will temporarily blur the vision after application. Temporary or permanent lacrimal punctal occlusion may give symptomatic relief by preventing drainage and side shields on spectacles or lateral tarsorrhaphy may help by preventing evaporation of tears.

Watery eyes

Watering of the eyes is a frequent occurrence in any eye disease and is due to excess production of tear fluid from the lacrimal gland. There is reflex watering of the eyes (lacrimation) in any inflammatory condition such as a corneal foreign body, iritis, acute glaucoma and injury, mediated through the trigeminal nerve (Vth cranial nerve). Physiological watering of the eyes may occur in particularly sensitive individuals in bright light or cold wind and also in emotional moments of sadness or laughter.

Eyelid disease causing malpositioning of the lacrimal puncta and any obstruction in the lacrimal passageways will cause overflow of tears on to the cheek (**epiphora**). Whenever watering of the eye or eyes occurs treatment should be directed to the cause. Particular features to note when examining the lacrimal apparatus are the position and opening of the puncta, obvious overspill of tears on to the cheek, the position of the eyelids and any evidence of swelling over the lacrimal gland (lateral part of upper eyelid) or over the lacrimal sac (side of the nose). The orbicularis oculi muscle aids normal drainage of tears by forcing tears into the lacrimal sac during blinking ('lacrimal pump'). Loss of this lacrimal pump in VIIth nerve palsy frequently results in epiphora.

It is important to remember that epiphora in infants may be the only symptom of congenital glaucoma (see Chapter 10).

PUNCTUM AND CANALICULUS OBSTRUCTION

Congenital absence or incomplete development of the punctum and canaliculus is rare and causes the same symptoms as a congenitally obstructed nasolacrimal duct, namely watering and stickiness of the eye. More commonly punctum and canaliculus obstructions arise as a result of chronic conjunctivitis (especially herpes simplex and Chlamydia) or as an accompaniment of mucocutaneous disease (pemphigus, ocular pemphigoid, Stevens–Johnson syndrome). Trauma to the lacrimal canalicula is not uncommon and may lead to epiphora.

Treatment

Symptomatic epiphora arising from punctal stenosis may be relieved by simple punctal dilatation or surgical enlargement. Canalicular blockage is more challenging and repair usually consists of an extensive canaliculus reconstruction operation.

CONGENITAL NASOLACRIMAL DUCT OBSTRUCTION

See Chapter 14.

ADULT NASOLACRIMAL DUCT OBSTRUCTION

Long-standing watering of the eyes in the elderly patient is a common occurrence. It may be due to obstruction of the nasolacrimal duct caused by chronic infection (chronic dacrocystitis) or involutional stenosis. The main symptom experienced by the patient is overspill of tears onto the cheeks especially in cold winds. Certain patients complain of a persistent mucous discharge. There are no characteristic signs but it is important to note that the lids and puncta are anatomically normal and the absence of any inflammation or swelling. The diagnosis may be confirmed by gently syringing saline through the lower punctum and canaliculus after instillation of local anaesthetic drops (amethocaine or benoxinate). If the patient can feel saline in his nasopharynx then the lacrimal passageway must be clear; if not and it returns via the upper punctum then this indicates obstruction of the nasolacrimal duct (Fig. 6.3).

Treatment

A mild degree of watering due to nasolacrimal duct obstruction in the elderly is best left untreated. A simple explanation of this harmless condition will allay the anxiety of patients and allow them to accept this minor disability once the diagnosis has been made.

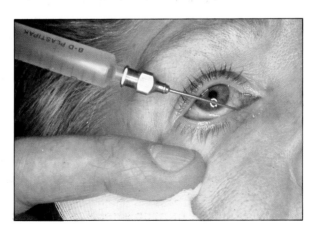

Figure 6.3
Syringing the nasolacrimal duct

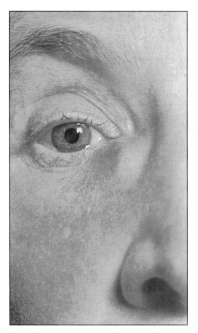

Figure 6.4
Acute dacryocystitis

Severe watering of the eyes can be very distressing, producing erythema and dryness of the skin of the cheeks with blurring of vision. Treatment in these circumstances is the operation of dacryocystorhinostomy, a surgical procedure that bypasses the obstructed nasolacrimal duct by anastomosing the mucosa lining the lacrimal sac with that of the nasal passages through an opening fashioned in the bone of the lateral wall of the nose. This may be performed either externally through the skin or endonasally.

ACUTE DACRYOCYSTITIS

Acute infection of the lacrimal sac will almost always occur where there is pre-existing chronic obstruction or infection. Consequently there is often a long history of watering of the eye prior to the acute event.

The symptom of acute dacryocystitis is rapid onset of a painful swelling at the side of the nose near the inner canthus of the eye. The characteristic sign is a reddened, tender, tense swelling between the side of the nose and just below the inner canthus. Watering and discharge from the eye usually occurs (Fig. 6.4).

Treatment

Systemic antibiotics are required (e.g. ampicillin or flucloxacillin 250 mg four times a day for 7 days). When the acute inflammation has subsided a mucocoele (collection of mucus in the dilated lacrimal sac) may remain with constant regurgitation of mucus upwards into the conjunctiva. Recurrent dacryocystitis or mucocoele usually requires dacryocystorhinostomy to effect a permanent cure.

Lacrimal gland disorders

DACRYOADENITIS

Dacryoadenitis is inflammation of the lacrimal gland. The symptoms are swelling and tenderness of the lateral aspect of the upper eyelid often with epiphora. The signs are a tender swelling on the lateral aspect of the upper eyelid with

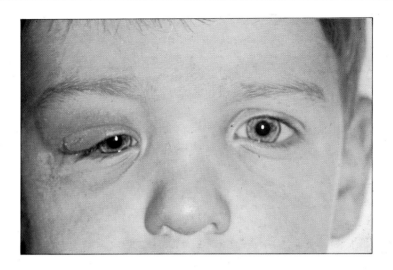

Figure 6.5
Acute dacryoadenitis

erythema of the overlying skin. Gently raising the upper eyelid will reveal the enlarged, sometimes discharging, lacrimal gland. The pre-auricular lymph nodes may also be enlarged (Figs 6.5 and 6.6).

Dacryoadenitis is most common in young people and may be caused by:

- **Acute infections**. Those caused by staphylococci or haemophilus influenzae bacteria may be blood-borne but may also be introduced by injuries to the lacrimal gland. Infective dacryoadenitis may lead to orbital cellulitis if not promptly treated.

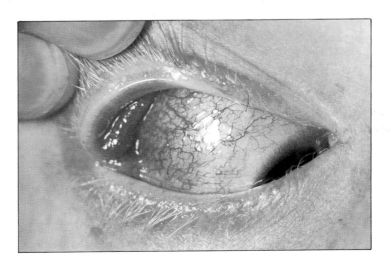

Figure 6.6
Inflamed lacrimal gland

- **Chronic infections**. These may be tubercular in origin and in these patients there may be other signs (e.g. pulmonary tuberculosis).
- **Mumps**. This is a viral infection that occurs mainly in children causing enlargement of the lacrimal and salivary glands and usually resolving over a few days. Infectious mononucleosis (Epstein–Barr virus) may cause a similar transient dacryoadenitis.
- **Sarcoidosis**. This frequently involves the lacrimal glands causing a chronic dacryoadenitis. There may be other signs of sarcoidosis such as enlarged salivary glands, pulmonary and skin changes.

Treatment

The treatment of dacryoadenitis is directed at the cause in each case. Where a precise diagnosis of a chronic dacryoadenitis is not possible with clinical evidence alone, it is sometimes necessary to perform a surgical biopsy of the enlarged gland for microscopic examination.

NEOPLASMS OF THE LACRIMAL GLAND

Tumours of the lacrimal gland are uncommon and occur mainly in the middle-aged. The main clinical feature is progressive enlargement of the gland which can be felt through the upper eyelid as a hard irregular mass. This occurs gradually over several months and as a result the eye becomes proptosed, often with downward displacement.

The majority of lacrimal gland neoplasms are mixed tumours, adenocarcinomas or lymphomas.

Mixed tumours (pleomorphic adenoma), so called because they contain mesenchymal and epithelial elements, affect middle-aged people who present with a long history of a painless, slowly enlarging mass or proptosis. Treatment is by local surgical excision.

Adenoid cystic carcinoma is the commonest and most aggressive adenocarcinoma affecting the lacrimal gland. This also usually presents in middle age but the history of gland swelling is shorter (over a few weeks) and there is often associated pain due to bony destruction. Treatment is by radiotherapy, or radical surgical excision for the locally invasive tumours (Fig. 6.7).

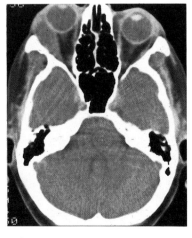

Figure 6.7
CT scan of head: note proptosis of left eye and tumour in lateral and posterior orbit (lacrimal gland adenoid cystic carcinoma)

Lymphoma or lymphosarcoma of the lacrimal gland is usually associated with widespread reticulosis. Treatment is usually by radiotherapy or chemotherapy.

7 Inflamed eyes

Anatomy

The anterior portion of the eye has two separate blood supplies, namely the conjunctival and ciliary vessels. The conjunctival arteries are numerous small branches from the eyelid arterial arcades and the anterior ciliary arteries. They have numerous corresponding veins providing venous blood drainage. The anterior ciliary arteries are continuations of the paired arteries running forwards in the four rectus muscles and they can easily be seen in normal eyes. They penetrate the sclera to supply blood to the ciliary body and iris, also sending off small branches that join the conjunctival vessels. Venous drainage is by similar ciliary veins.

The two long posterior ciliary arteries are branches of the ophthalmic artery. They penetrate the sclera either side of the optic nerve before passing forwards in the space between choroid and sclera to anastomose with the anterior ciliary

Figures 7.1 a and b
Blood supply to anterior portion of eye and eyelids

(a)

(b)

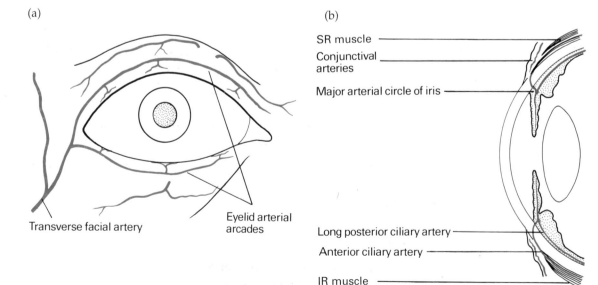

Transverse facial artery

Eyelid arterial arcades

SR muscle

Conjunctival arteries

Major arterial circle of iris

Long posterior ciliary artery

Anterior ciliary artery

IR muscle

arteries in the ciliary body and form the major arterial circle of the iris (Figs 7.1 a and b).

Conditions of the anterior segment and cornea (iritis, acute glaucoma, keratitis) cause dilatation of the ciliary vessels and this is called **ciliary hyperaemia or injection**. Clinically this appears as redness of the eye which is most intense around the cornea (circumcorneal or limbal) becoming less intense at the periphery of the conjunctiva.

Conditions of the conjunctiva (conjunctivitis) cause dilatation of the conjunctival vessels, called **conjunctival hyperaemia or injection**. Clinically this appears as redness which is most marked over the tarsal and peripheral bulbar conjunctiva with relative sparing around the cornea.

Conditions causing red eye will be discussed under the following headings:

- Conjunctivitis
- Keratitis
- Iritis
- Acute glaucoma
- Other conditions. — Trauma
  Subconjunctival haemorrhage
  Corneal Ulceration
  Scleritis

Conjunctivitis

Inflammation of the conjunctiva, a mucous membrane, is called conjunctivitis.

Causes

- Bacterial infections especially staphylococcus, haemophilus influenzae, streptococcus and Chlamydia
- Viral infections especially herpes simplex and adenovirus
- Allergy
- Trauma especially chemicals and ultraviolet energy irradiation (see Chapter 9)
- Dry eyes (conjunctivitis sicca) due to lack of tear secretion (see Chapter 6)
- Blepharitis (see Chapter 5).

Symptoms

- Sensation of grittiness or 'sandy' feeling
- Watery or purulent discharge

- Reddened appearance of the eyes
- In severe cases the eyelids may be swollen
- Itching–suggests allergic conjunctivitis.

Signs

- Conjunctival hyperaemia (Fig. 7.2)
- Mucus discharge on the conjunctiva and lids with crusting of the eyelashes
- Eyelid swelling
- Normal visual acuity
- Pre-auricular lymphadenopathy often accompanies viral conjunctivitis.

Treatment

Swabs are taken for bacteriology and virology and cell scrapings for Chlamydia if the condition is severe or chronic, or the diagnosis uncertain. Lid cleaning to remove the crusts on the eyelids every few hours using cotton wool soaked in boiled tepid water is comforting.

With bacterial infections antibiotic eye drops are instilled initially every 2 hours. Antibiotic ointment may also be used at night. Chloramphenicol (Chloromycetin) is the most widely used topical therapy and is only changed if the culture shows the bacterium is not sensitive. Bacterial conjunctivitis usually settles within 3–4 days on antibiotic drops. If the

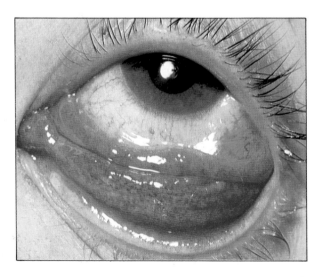

Figure 7.2
Acute conjunctivitis

situation is not improving on an adequate therapeutic regimen then infection with either Chlamydia or a virus should be considered.

In conjunctivitis caused by adenovirus, herpes or Chlamydia trachomatis, pre-auricular lymphadenopathy and conjunctival follicles are common. Follicles are fine (about 1 mm), rounded collections of lymphoid tissue, mostly in the inferior conjunctival fornix.

Chlamydia infections should be diagnosed by taking the appropriate swabs and a genitourinary opinion is often required. Treatment requires systemic tetracycline or erythromycin (see Chapter 15).

Viral conjunctivitis is extremely difficult to treat and may persist for many weeks. Certain viral infections, particularly adenovirus are extremely contagious, and appropriate advice needs to be given to avoid spread by direct contact. If the vision is affected specialist advice and treatment should be sought.

ALLERGIC CONJUNCTIVITIS

Allergic conjunctivitis may occur as an acute episode in response to a particular antigen (e.g. cat hair), it may occur seasonally for a few months a year in patients with pollen allergy (hay fever) or it may be a chronic problem, often in children or young adults with other atopic diseases such as asthma or eczema.

Symptoms and signs

- Ocular discomfort, photophobia and itching
- Conjunctival hyperaemia
- The characteristic sign is that of papillae on the tarsal conjunctiva on eversion of the upper eyelid. In children with chronic allergic conjunctivitis (vernal conjunctivitis) these papillae are often flat-topped and large, known as cobblestones (Fig. 7.3).

Treatment

Oral and topical antihistamines (e.g. Otrivine drops) may be useful for relieving symptoms in hay fever and acute allergic conjunctivitis respectively. Mast cell stabilisers such as

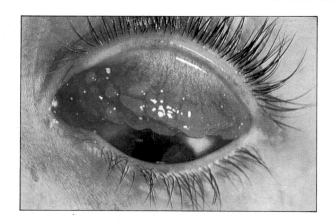

Figure 7.3
Vernal conjunctivitis showing papillae on upper tarsal conjunctiva

Opticrom, Alomide or Rapitil, used for a prolonged period will often reduce the frequency of acute exacerbations of a chronic or seasonal allergic conjunctivitis.

Topical steroid drops may have to be considered in severe cases. These should only be used under specialist supervision.

Keratitis

This term covers any inflammation of the cornea. Since the cornea is exposed constantly during the waking day it is not surprising that externally induced infection occurs fairly commonly.

Keratitis initially produces a localised oedema of the cornea, rapidly followed by infiltration of inflammatory cells, hence the invariable sign of a localised corneal opacity. With long-standing keratitis, vascularisation of the cornea and abscess formation occurs (Fig. 7.4).

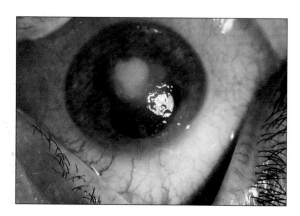

Figure 7.4
Corneal abscess: note white area of abscess of inflammatory cells. (Courtesy of the Western Ophthalmic Hospital)

Organisms causing keratitis are usually bacteria (such as staphylococci, streptococci) or viruses (such as herpes simplex, adenovirus and herpes zoster). Acanthamoeba is a protozoan and is an increasingly common cause of keratitis in soft contact lens wearers.

Symptoms

- Rapid blurring of vision in one, or both, eye(s)
- Redness of the eye
- Aching pain in the eye
- Photophobia
- Watering of the eye.

Signs

- Reduced visual acuity
- Ciliary vessel hyperaemia
- Swelling of eyelids
- Localised corneal opacity. This is the most important and distinctive sign of keratitis, and the appearance of the localised corneal opacity depends on the cause of the keratitis. Infective keratitis is usually associated with an epithelial defect overlying the corneal stromal opacity, and this stains with fluorescein (**corneal ulcer**).

HERPES SIMPLEX KERATITIS

There is a characteristic branching dendritic ulcer visible on the cornea. This may be more easily visualised by installation

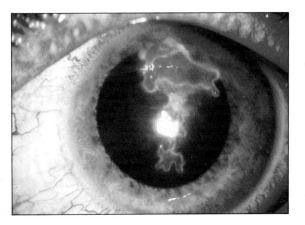

Figure 7.5
Dendritic ulcer of cornea (stained with fluorescein)

of fluorescein or rose bengal which stain the defective epithelium (Figs 7.5 and 7.6). The ulcer may progress to involve the deeper (stromal) layers of the cornea, in which case corneal opacification may develop (Fig. 7.7).

Treatment

A dendritic ulcer, or its deeper form, is treated with topical antiviral preparations most commonly acyclovir (Zovirax) 3% five times a day. This is usually required for a minimum of 10 days. Topical steroids may be needed to treat stromal keratitis but this should only be undertaken by specialists.

It should be emphasised that, in a patient with a uniocular red eye a diagnosis of herpes simplex should always be considered, and topical steroids should never be used unless herpes infection has been ruled out. If steroids are used

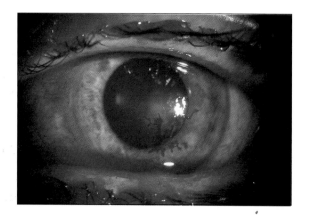

Figure 7.6
Dendritic ulcer of cornea (stained with rose bengal)

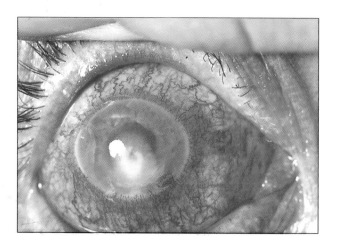

Figure 7.7
Deep stromal keratitis in herpes simplex

inadvertently the viral infection may run riot causing extensive corneal scarring.

ADENOVIRUS KERATITIS

Occasionally a severe adenovirus conjunctivitis may cause a keratitis. This may be associated with ocular pain and variable reduction in vision. Keratitis is recognised as numerous small, circular, corneal stromal opacities in a patient with intense follicular conjunctivitis (Fig. 7.8).

Treatment

There is no specific antiviral treatment. Topical antibiotics are usually given to prevent secondary bacterial infection. In severe cases where the keratitis has seriously and significantly reduced vision topical steroid therapy may also be indicated. This must be done under specialist supervision.

ACANTHAMOEBA KERATITIS

This is a serious infection associated with soft contact lens wear and inadequate lens hygiene, and can be prevented by proper lens cleaning. It is difficult to diagnose and requires prolonged specialist treatment.

HERPES ZOSTER OPHTHALMICUS

Herpes zoster ophthalmicus (HZO) is the name given to shingles affecting the ophthalmic division of the trigeminal

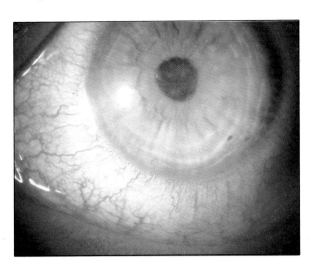

Figure 7.8
Adenovirus keratitis showing spot corneal opacities and ciliary hyperaemia

nerve. It occurs with reactivation of the varicella virus which had previously laid dormant in the trigeminal nerve ganglion from an original chickenpox infection. Once reactivated the varicella virus travels down the ophthalmic nerve to the nerve endings. It is more common in the elderly and those with reduced immunity and is seen after trauma (particularly injection of the trigeminal ganglion). The signs are preceded by prodromal 'flu-like illness. As ocular structures are supplied by the same nerve eye complications may occur.

Signs and symptoms

There is characteristically a unilateral skin rash over the forehead and usually down the side of the nose which corresponds to the skin distribution of the ophthalmic division of the trigeminal nerve. Vesicles develop which start to crust after about a week (Fig. 7.9). Skin scarring may develop. Patients often complain of pain over the affected dermatome which may persist long after the skin lesions have resolved. This **post-herpetic neuralgia** may be extremely debilitating and is very difficult to treat.

Ocular complications

- Swelling and lid scarring
- Red eye due to conjunctivitis, keratitis or uveitis

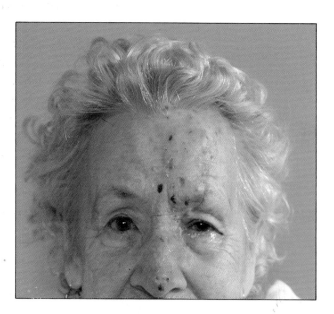

Figure 7.9
Herpes zoster ophthalmicus

- Glaucoma may develop as a result of uveitis, or as a response to the topical steroid therapy
- Following HZO the cornea may be left markedly or completely anaesthetic. As normal corneal sensation is required to maintain a healthy ocular surface affected patients may develop corneal damage and ulceration (neuropathic keratitis)
- Extraocular muscle palsies and optic neuritis may occur.

Treatment

If diagnosed within the first 48 hours, systemic treatment with an antiviral should be started (such as acyclovir). Systemic treatment is reported to halt vesiculation, speed healing and reduce post-herpetic neuralgia. Acyclovir cream applied to the skin vesicles very early in the course of the disease may be helpful.

Ocular complications may require treatment with topical acyclovir and/or steroids under specialist supervision.

Iritis

The iris, ciliary body and choroid are one continuous layer called the uveal tract and because of their vascularity, intraocular inflammation predominates in these structures.

Inflammation of the iris (iritis) invariably occurs with that of the ciliary body (cyclitis) so the terms iritis, iridocyclitis and anterior uveitis are interchangeable for practical purposes. The inflammation within iris tissues is likely to be due to an antigen–antibody reaction in a previously sensitised iris. The seronegative arthropathies (such as Still's disease, Reiter's disease and Behçet's disease in particular) are associated with iritis. Histocompatibility antigens (HLA) have been associated with iritis, especially HLA-B27. Precisely how this mechanism occurs is not fully understood, but does explain the recurrent nature of iritis. The known conditions associated with iritis are:

- Sarcoidosis
- Ankylosing spondylitis
- Reiter's disease
- Still's disease (juvenile rheumatoid arthritis) in children

- Behçet's disease (see Chapter 15)
- Tuberculosis
- Syphilis
- Leprosy
- Sympathetic uveitis: an autoimmune inflammatory reaction that may occur in both eyes after one eye has had exposure of uveal tissue following ocular surgery or penetrating trauma. Because of this risk it is often advised that severely traumatised eyes should be enucleated within 10–14 days of injury to prevent the onset of sympathetic uveitis in the remaining good eye.

Investigations of selected patients with iritis might include full blood count, angiotensin converting enzyme assay, X-rays of sacroiliac joints and chest, serological tests for syphilis, HLA typing, Mantoux testing and other investigations as indicated. It should be noted that the cause of iritis is seldom established.

Symptoms

- Rapid blurring of vision in one, or both, eye(s) over hours or days
- Redness of the eye
- Aching pain in the eye
- Photophobia
- Watering of the eye.

Signs

- Reduced visual acuity
- Ciliary vessel hyperaemia
- Pupil constriction: because of inflammatory spasm of the iris sphincter muscle
- Flare and cells in the anterior chamber: protein exudate and inflammatory cells respectively may be seen on the slit lamp with a focused light in the anterior chamber (Fig. 7.10). If the inflammation is very severe there may be a fluid level of white cells seen called a **hypopyon**
- Keratitic precipitates (KP): the inflammatory cells circulating in the aqueous may be deposited on the posterior surface of the cornea in blobs (Fig. 7.11)
- Pupil irregularity: **posterior synechiae** are adhesions

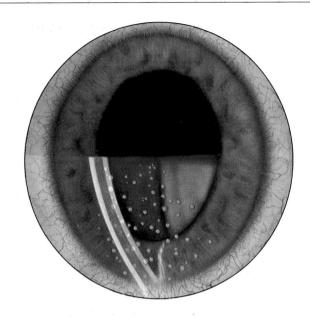

Figure 7.10
Painting of flare and keratitic precipitates (KP) on posterior corneal surface in iritis

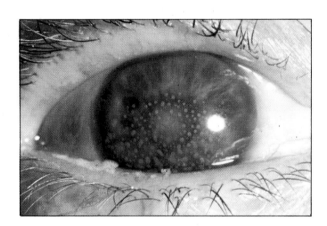

Figure 7.11
Extensive KP in iritis

between the iris and lens and may lead to a secondary glaucoma (Fig. 7.12)

- Swelling of the eyelids.

Treatment

Topical steroid therapy usually starting with steroid drops every 2 hours. There is a range of strength of steroids ranging from Prednisolone Forte as the strongest through dexamethasone (Maxidex), Betnesol and Predsol to the weakest, FML. The choice of appropriate steroid strength depends on the severity of the iritis.

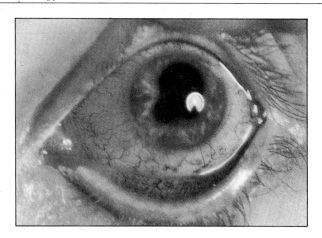

Figure 7.12
Posterior synechiae in iritis

Mydriatic eye drops such as cyclopentolate 1% or atropine 1% are used 1–3 times per day to reduce the discomfort caused by iris spasm and to prevent the formation of posterior synechiae.

Treatment is slowly tapered off as the anterior chamber activity settles. The intraocular pressure should be regularly monitored to check for secondary glaucoma in any patient on topical steroid therapy. Any underlying disease should receive specific treatment as required.

Acute glaucoma

See Chapter 10 on glaucoma.

Other causes

PTERYGIUM

Exposure to hot, dry and dusty conditions in many parts of the world e.g. India, Africa and Australia, causes a thickening and ingrowth of palpebral conjunctiva on to the cornea (Fig. 7.13).

Treatment

This usually requires no treatment but if growth continues over the cornea threatening the visual axis or is considered cosmetically unacceptable surgical removal is indicated.

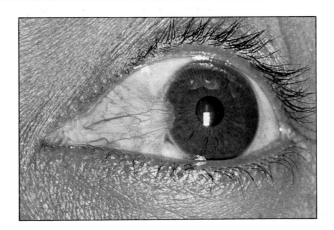

Figure 7.13
Pterygium

A pterygium may become inflamed requiring treatment with topical steroids. Topical lubrication may be helpful to prevent irritation.

EPISCLERITIS

Presents as a localised, slightly raised area of hyperaemia of episcleral vessels close to the corneal margin, occasionally centred around a nodule. It causes minor discomfort only. The cause is unknown and recurrence is frequent (Fig. 7.14).

Treatment

Usually settles without treatment but a short course of a weak topical steroid may be helpful.

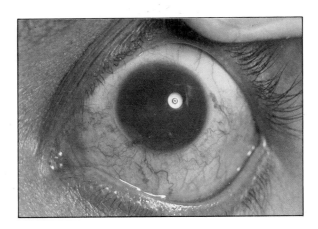

Figure 7.14
Episcleritis

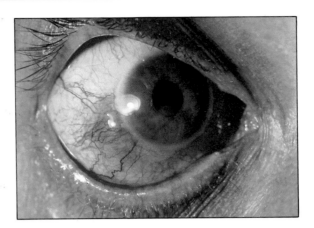

Figure 7.15
Scleritis

SCLERITIS

This is an uncommon but potentially serious eye disorder. It presents with a dull, deep, aching pain, which may be severe. There is intense localised ciliary hyperaemia of one section of the eye which may spread to involve the whole sclera. It is associated with rheumatoid arthritis, systemic lupus and polyarteritis nodosa (Fig. 7.15).

Treatment

Non-steroidal anti-inflammatories such as Froben 50 mg t.d.s. Systemic steroids may be required in severe cases.

SUMMARY OF SYMPTOMS AND SIGNS OF CAUSES OF RED EYES

	Symptoms	*Signs*
Conjunctivitis	Red eyes Bilateral (usually) Gritty feeling Stickiness	Conjunctival hyperaemia Swollen eyelids Mucoid discharge
Keratitis	Red eye Unilateral (usually) Lacrimation Photophobia Blurred vision Pain	Reduced vision Ciliary injection Localised corneal opacification
Iritis	Red eye Unilateral (usually) Lacrimation Photophobia Blurred vision Pain	Reduced vision Ciliary injection Constricted pupil Flare in anterior chamber Keratitic precipitates
Acute glaucoma	Red eye Unilateral (usually) Lacrimation Photophobia Blurred vision Pain Haloes	Reduced vision Ciliary injection Corneal oedema (cloudy) Pupil mid-dilated and oval Raised ocular tension

8 Eye injuries and first aid

Eye injuries are dramatic and invariably produce considerable emotional upset for the patient. Whenever possible advice should be provided to prevent them occurring in industrial and social environments.

Ocular injuries will be discussed under the following headings:

- Prevention of eye injuries
- First aid equipment
- Orbital injuries
- Eyelid injuries
- Eye injuries.

Prevention of eye injuries

Industry and building

Adequate protective spectacles or visors should be worn to prevent foreign body, irradiation (especially ultraviolet and infrared radiation) and chemical injuries to the eyes.

Transport

The wearing of a seat belt prevents most of the severe eye injuries caused by an unrestrained occupant being thrown through the windscreen. Seat belts must be worn by all drivers and front seat passengers and used if fitted by back seat passengers. Children should always be harnessed in an appropriate car seat. Laminated rather than toughened glass windscreens are now used in most motor vehicles as this markedly reduces splintering. Some cars are fitted with driver and front passenger airbags which prevent severe facial injury from hitting the steering wheel or dashboard in the event of a collision.

Sports

Sports are now an important cause of serious eye damage, especially football and racket sports. These injuries are commonest in 10- to 19-year-old males. Many of these injuries could be reduced or prevented by wearing adequate eye protection (Fig. 8.1).

Sports injuries can be caused by blunt trauma from flying objects such as balls, by parts of the body such as elbows, or by being hit with rackets or sticks. Sharp injuries can be caused by the breakage of glass spectacle lenses, and patients should be advised to use plastic spectacle lenses or contact lenses when playing sport rather than spectacles with glass lenses. Radiation injury can occur by exposure to ultraviolet light when skiing and engaging in water sports.

Other occasions

The sun should never be looked at directly with or without tinted spectacles because of the risk of retinal (macular) burns. This applies especially at the time of the sun's eclipse.

Do-it-yourself handymen should use protective goggles or spectacles (polycarbonate) when using power drills or heavy hammers.

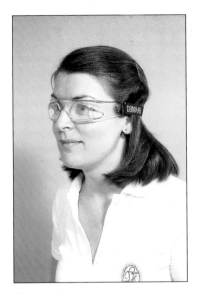

Figure 8.1
Protective eyewear for racket sports

First aid equipment

A simple first aid kit should contain the following (Fig. 8.2):

* Torch for illumination
* Local anaesthetic to anaesthetise the superficial cornea and conjunctiva e.g. amethocaine, benoxinate or proxymetacaine
* Fluorescein drops or strips to detect corneal abrasions; fluorescein stains areas of epithelial loss and this is particularly obvious if viewed using a blue light
* Cotton buds for removing superficial foreign bodies and for everting the eyelid
* Antibiotic eye ointment or drops, e.g. Chloromycetin or Fucithalmic

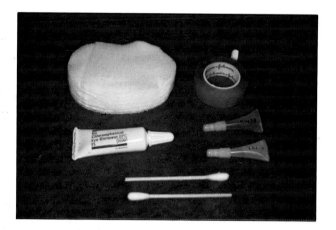

Figure 8.2
Simple essentials for eye first aid

- Eye pads
- Tape for holding eye pad in place, e.g. Micropore, Transpore.

Single-dose ampoules of fluorescein and antibiotic are particularly suitable as they provide a supply of sterile eye drops which can be discarded after use.

Orbital injuries

A severe concussion blow to the orbital region by a heavy object or fist usually causes considerable periorbital swelling and bruising. This may be so extensive that it is difficult to open the eyelids, even forcibly, to examine the eye (Fig. 8.3).

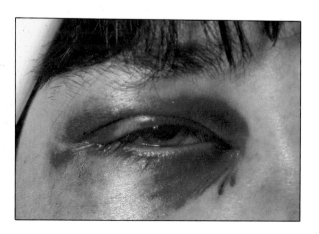

Figure 8.3
Periorbital and subconjunctival haemorrhage

Bleeding into the orbit from a blow may cause subconjunctival haemorrhage, protrusion of the eye (proptosis), and if severe may impair vision due to optic nerve compression by the haematoma (retrobulbar haemorrhage). Any patient who has sustained blunt trauma to the eye such that the lids cannot be opened to allow ocular examination and visual acuity assessment or who has marked proptosis or reduced vision should be referred for urgent ophthalmological assessment.

'Blow out' fractures of the orbital floor should be suspected whenever there is any severe periorbital swelling and bruising with a history of a blow or other trauma to the area. The fracture is a break in the floor of the orbit and can be recognised clinically by the following signs:

- Enophthalmos, due to soft orbital tissues prolapsing through the fractured orbital floor causing the eye to sink back in the orbit
- Diplopia and restricted eye movement on looking upwards and downwards, either because of tethering of the inferior rectus muscle in the fracture line or bruising of the inferior rectus muscle
- Anaesthesia of the skin of the lower eyelid and cheek because of damage to the infraorbital nerve
- Bruising and sometimes surgical emphysema of the eyelids due to escape of air from associated fractures of the ethmoid sinuses.

A thorough eye examination should be conducted because up to 10 per cent of patients with blow out fractures of the orbit will have sustained ocular damage. A plain X-ray of the orbit may not clearly demonstrate a small floor fracture and if there is any doubt the patient should have a CT scan. Providing damage to the eye itself has not taken place the patient is observed to allow settling of the periorbital bruising, and very frequently the traumatised inferior rectus muscle function improves in 7–10 days. Only if handicapping diplopia and significant enophthalmos is still present a few weeks after the injury is it necessary to operate to release the tethered inferior rectus muscle and repair the orbital floor fracture.

Eyelid injuries

Lacerations of the eyelid from sharp objects should be cleaned and sutured as soon as possible. It is important that the tissue layers are repaired very carefully to prevent distortion of the eyelids. Any laceration on the medial quarter of the lower eyelid should receive particular attention because of the danger of severance of the lower canaliculus; this can damage tear drainage leading to epiphora.

Eye injuries

SUBCONJUNCTIVAL HAEMORRHAGE

Bleeding into the subconjunctival tissue can occur from even a trivial injury. The bright red appearance localised to one area of the conjunctiva is characteristic. No treatment is required provided there is no other injured tissue. The haemorrhage spontaneously resolves over about 10–14 days (Fig. 8.3). Dense, widespread subconjunctival haemorrhage in association with blunt trauma may indicate the possibility of an associated orbital haemorrhage. Some patients develop spontaneous subconjunctival haemorrhage which may be associated with systemic hypertension.

CONJUNCTIVAL AND CORNEAL FOREIGN BODIES

Small particles may blow onto the surface of the eye and cause an intense pricking sensation, redness and watering of the eye. Metallic corneal foreign bodies are common when using a grinding machine without protective spectacles. With a good light, and everting the upper eyelid, the foreign body can be detected on the surface of the cornea or conjunctiva (Fig. 8.4).

Treatment

Instil local anaesthetic drops and remove foreign body gently with cotton bud. If the foreign body is iron there may be a residual 'rust ring' on the cornea following removal. There is usually a small corneal abrasion following removal of a corneal foreign body which should be treated as described below.

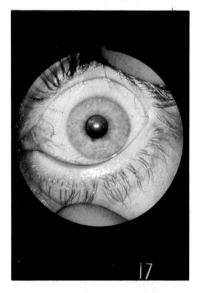

Figure 8.4
Corneal foreign body

A rust ring may need to be left to 'soften' for 2 days before it can be removed by the ophthalmologist.

Eversion of the eyelid

This simple technique should be employed whenever a subtarsal foreign body is suspected of being lodged under the upper lid. The patient is asked to look down, the cotton bud handle is placed horizontally on the upper eyelid, the eyelashes held and the eyelid gently turned over the cotton bud handle (Figs 8.5 a and b). The foreign body can then gently be wiped away with the cotton bud.

CORNEAL ABRASIONS

The surface corneal epithelium may be sloughed off by a glancing blow to the eye from an object such as a fingernail or twig. Exposure to ultraviolet light (as in arc welders or 'arc

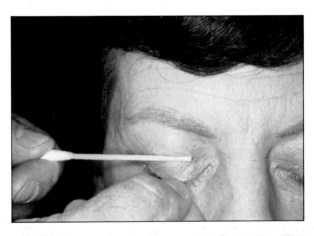

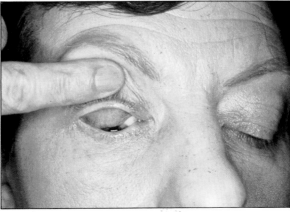

(b)

Figure 8.5 a and b
Eversion of upper eyelid

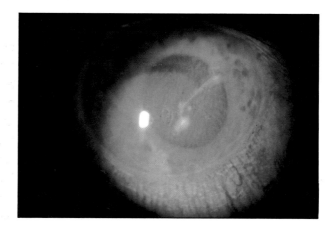

Figure 8.6
Corneal abrasion stained with
fluorescein

eye') produces multiple tiny corneal abrasions and severe pain in both eyes.

Whatever the cause the eye or eyes are very painful watery, red and photophobic. The diagnosis may be readily made by using fluorescein to detect the corneal abrasion or abrasions (Fig. 8.6).

Treatment

Check that no foreign body is still present in the eye. Antibiotic ointment is instilled into the eye and an eye pad is applied to keep the eye closed for 12–24 hours. Following removal of the eye pad antibiotic drops or ointment are applied to the eye for about 5 days. Most corneal abrasions are healed within 48–72 hours.

Recurrent corneal erosion is the name given to a repeated painful eye weeks or months after the original injury and usually presents in the early morning after awakening. It is due to recurrent breakdown of the originally damaged corneal epithelium and mimics the signs and symptoms of the original abrasion. It is thought to occur because the recently healed area of epithelium is not firmly anchored to the deeper layers of the cornea, rendering it liable to adhere to the upper lid during sleep and to tear off on eye opening. When such recurrent abrasions occur lubricating ointment such as Lacrilube or Simple eye ointment instilled at night may prevent the episodes.

CHEMICAL INJURIES

Whenever chemicals of any description are splashed into the eyes immediate immersion of the eyes in water is vital and washing the eyes liberally (preferably in running water) should be continued for as long as 20 minutes. In hospital this is done after instillation of local anaesthetic and is continued until the ocular tear film achieves a normal pH. The eyelids should be everted and the fornix examined for any particulate matter that may still be trapped. Specialist treatment should then be sought at once. Alkali injuries are particularly devastating and extreme care, including the use of protective goggles, should be taken when handling these substances.

HYPHAEMA (HAEMORRHAGE INTO THE ANTERIOR CHAMBER)

A concussion injury to the eye from a blow for example from a fist, explosion or any heavy object, may cause haemorrhage into the anterior chamber (between the cornea and iris) from the rupture of iris blood vessels.

There is immediate severe pain and blurring of vision and in a few minutes the eye becomes hyperaemic. Examination reveals blood in the anterior chamber which forms a 'fluid level' and obscures the view of the iris and pupil (Fig. 8.7). Rest in bed in hospital or home is necessary because of the danger of secondary haemorrhage into the anterior chamber. This secondary haemorrhage may be a good deal more severe than the original one and can cause secondary glaucoma.

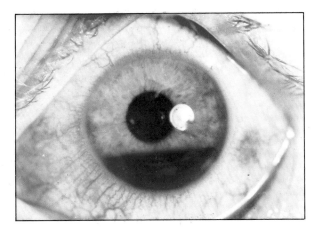

Figure 8.7
Hyphaema

Such a secondary haemorrhage usually occurs within 10 days of the injury.

Most hyphaemas slowly absorb over about 7 days with rest. Full inspection of the retina through the dilated pupil is essential once the hyphaema has cleared to detect any associated retinal damage.

IRIS DISINSERTION (IRIDODIALYSIS)

The periphery of the iris is its weakest part and a concussion injury may cause tearing of the iris root giving an iridodialysis. The appearance is like an extra peripheral 'pupil' (Fig. 8.8). An iridodialysis will be accompanied by a hyphaema at the time of the injury. The patient should have long-term follow up because of the risk of secondary glaucoma due to damage to the anterior chamber drainage angle.

LENS SUBLUXATION

Any severe blow to the eye may cause displacement of the lens by rupturing the lens suspensory fibres. The lens may be displaced backwards into the vitreous (posterior subluxation or dislocation) or forwards into the anterior chamber (anterior subluxation or dislocation). It can be recognised by the displacement of the lens in the pupil and by the tremulousness of the iris (iridodonesis) (Fig. 8.9).

Lens subluxation requires long-term specialist supervision because of the high risk of later secondary glaucoma and cataract formation.

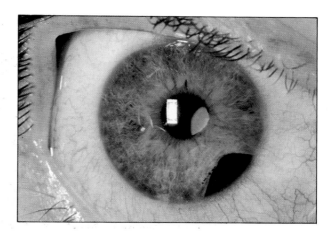

Figure 8.8
Iridodialysis

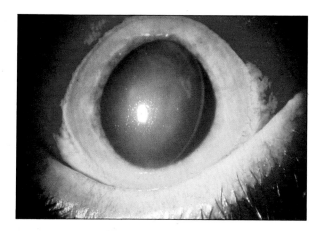

Figure 8.9
Subluxated lens

INTRAOCULAR FOREIGN BODIES

For a foreign body to penetrate the cornea or sclera and enter the eye it must be travelling at a very high velocity. Most are particles of metal and result from explosions, machinery, power tools or from using a hammer and metal chisel. The patient normally experiences a foreign body sensation as the particle strikes the eye but occasionally it enters unnoticed. Sudden loss of vision and pain are usual.

Careful examination will reveal the small corneal or scleral wound at the point of entry and the foreign body itself in the iris or further back in the vitreous or retina (Fig. 8.10). If the foreign body strikes the lens a cataract supervenes in a few hours. When an intraocular foreign body is suspected from the nature of the injury but none detected on examination an X-ray of the ocular regeion will usually identify a metallic

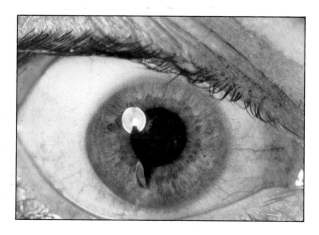

Figure 8.10
Metal foreign body embedded in the iris

foreign body (but not always a glass or plastic foreign body). If a non-metallic foreign body is suspected a CT scan should be undertaken.

Intraocular foreign bodies require surgical removal.

PENETRATING INJURIES

Any sharp object may penetrate the eye and cause sudden loss of vision, pain, watering and redness of the eye. Examples include knives, screwdrivers, darts, flying metal and car windscreen glass.

Aqueous immediately leaks out of a corneal wound but the iris plugs or prolapses into the wound which forms the classical signs of a distorted pupil, shallowed anterior chamber and a visible external iris prolapse in a hyperaemic eye (Fig. 8.11).

Immediate surgical repair of the wound and replacement of the iris is necessary.

RETINAL INJURIES AND RETINAL DETACHMENT

A penetrating or concussion injury to the eye may cause retinal damage. Other visible signs of injury such as bruising of the eyelids, iridodialysis and subluxated lens, should indicate the likelihood of accompanying retinal damage.

Retinal haemorrhage

Retinal haemorrhage following injury will be recognised with the ophthalmoscope providing there is no hyphaema

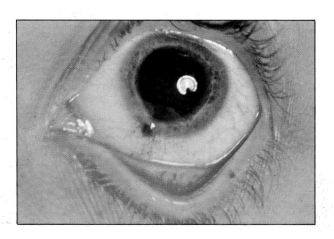

Figure 8.11
Perforating wound with prolapsed iris inferiorly

preventing a clear view. The patient gives a history of injury and notices sudden loss of vision at the time of the injury. The retinal haemorrhages and oedema (commotio retinae) are usually in the central area. No specific treatment is possible but slow resolution and some return of vision is likely over a period of several weeks or months.

Choroidal rupture

Splits in the choroid accompany severe concussion eye injuries with associated retinal haemorrhages and oedema. They may cause severe permanent visual impairment especially if a choroidal rupture underlies the central retina. The ophthalmoscopic appearance is that of whitish, circumscribed streaks in the central fundus. The whitish appearance is because the choroidal ruptures allow the underlying sclera to be visualised (Fig. 8.12).

Retinal detachment

A retinal detachment is usually associated with a break in the retina and any eye injury may cause this. The break may be a retinal tear or an area of disinsertion (retinal dialysis). A dialysis appears as a well-demarcated red area in the extreme periphery of the retina especially in the temporal region. A retinal detachment usually follows days or weeks after the injury.

If a retinal dialysis or tear can be diagnosed before fluid gets underneath the torn area and the retina detaches then the

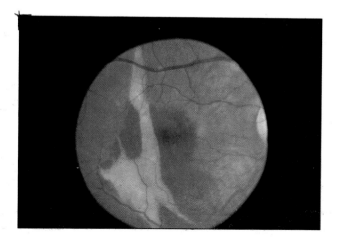

Figure 8.12
Choroidal tears and haemorrhage

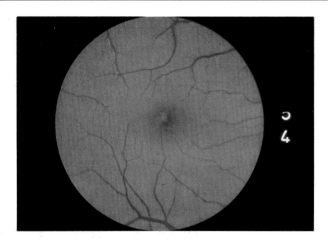

Figure 8.13
Solar macular burn

prognosis for vision is greatly improved. A retinal dialysis or tear can be 'sealed' by photocoagulation or cryotherapy; however once detachment has occurred a formal surgical procedure is required (see Chapter 11).

Solar retinal burns

Looking directly at the sun may result in a burn of the central retina. This is especially common at the time of the sun's eclipse when many people inadvisably do just this.

There is rapid loss of vision as a result of central retinal oedema which is replaced over several weeks by fine macular scarring in the form of pigmentary clumping. No treatment is effective (Fig. 8.13).

9 The lens

The crystalline lens is a transparent biconvex structure, approximately 10 mm in diameter and 4 mm at its thickest. It adds to the positive (convergent) refracting power of the cornea to focus parallel light rays on the retina. Embryologically it develops from ectoderm which accounts for the close relationship between many ectodermal (mainly skin) conditions and cataract (e.g. atopic eczema and scleroderma). The lens is held in position by fine suspensory zonule fibres which arise from the ciliary body and attach into the basement membrane capsule surrounding the lens (Fig. 9.1).

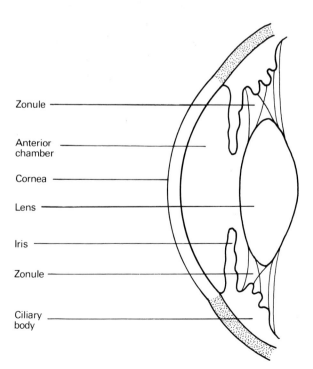

Zonule

Anterior chamber

Cornea

Lens

Iris

Zonule

Ciliary body

Figure 9.1
The lens in position in the anterior part of the eye

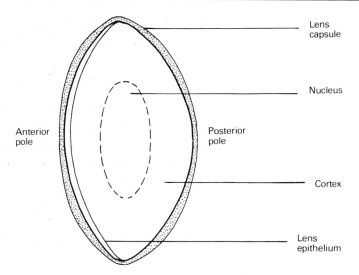

Figure 9.2
Section through a lens

Clinical slit lamp microscope examination of the lens reveals the characteristic transparent structure but various layers can be identified giving a clear observation of the laying down of the lens fibres from the embryo to birth (Fig. 9.2). The lens fibres are laid down from the epithelial layer lying at the most anterior portion of the lens and are arranged in such a precise and regular way that the lens is characteristically transparent.

Cataract

A cataract is any opacity of the crystalline lens; some are such minor variations in transparency that they do not affect vision whereas others may cause complete loss of lens transparency and blindness. Cataract is by far the commonest cause of blindness worldwide, accounting for some 16 million cases, all of which are potentially treatable. Examination with an ophthalmoscope reveals a reduced or absent red reflex for a generalised cataract and a black area within the red reflex for a localised lens opacity. A mature cataract prevents the visualisation of a red reflex and gives rise to the appearance of a white pupil or leukocoria.

Types of cataract are classified as follows:

- Developmental cataract
- Congenital cataract
- Senile cataract

- Cataract secondary to ocular disease
- Cataract associated with systemic disease.

DEVELOPMENTAL CATARACT

Developmental cataracts are minor opacities in the transparency of the lens and do not affect vision but are worthy of note in order to recognise that they are harmless when observed in patients being examined for other reasons. There are three types of developmental cataract that can be observed in a high proportion of the normal population and may be present at birth or develop in the first few years of life. It should be stressed that all three types (described below) are harmless.

Types of developmental cataract

- **Coronary lens opacities**. These are whitish or bluish finger-shaped opacities in the periphery of the lens cortex. They can usually only be seen with the pupil dilated.
- **Blue dot lens opacities**. Whitish or bluish dot opacities of varying size occur in the cortex of the lens in many people in the normal population (Fig. 9.3).
- **Dilacerated lens opacities**. This type of lens opacity is relatively unusual but appears as a striking bluish, fern leaf-like opacity in the lens cortex.

CONGENITAL CATARACT

Congenital cataracts are usually bilateral but unilateral ones

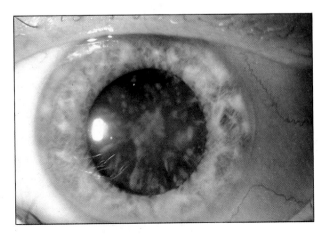

Figure 9.3
Blue dot and coronary developmental lens opacities; a more marked example than usual

may also occur. In the majority of infants the cause is not known, however aetiological factors include:

- Heredity
- Maternal infection (especially rubella), malnutrition or drugs ingestion
- Metabolic disorders (e.g. galactosaemia, hypocalcaemia)
- Chromosomal abnormalities (e.g Down's syndrome)
- Intraocular disease (e.g. uveitis, microphthalmos, retino-blastoma).

Symptoms

- The appearance of a white or grey pupil (leukocoria; see Chapter 14)
- A manifest strabismus (squint)
- Nystagmus.

Nystagmus is an indication of severe visual impairment and may vary from fine pendular to wide-ranging irregular eye movements. With unilateral cataract in particular, another associated cause should be looked for, e.g. retinoblastoma, toxoplasmosis and the presence of microphthalmos.

Types of congenital cataract

Congenital cataract may present with complete opacification of the lens or with opacification of a portion of the lens related to the stage of lens development when an insult was encountered. If a transient insult is encountered in early lens development the centre (embryological) nucleus is affected whereas if the insult occurs late in development a more peripheral nuclear or cortical lamellar layer may be involved. Numerous affected nuclear layers or a complete cataract suggests a prolonged insult during lens development.
There are three types of congenital cataract:

- **Nuclear cataract**. A central nuclear cataract suggests an insult early in lens development. It may appear as simple powder-like white spots in the nucleus of the lens (pulverulent cataract) or total opacification of the nucleus.
- **Lamellar (zonular) cataract**. This type of cataract derives its

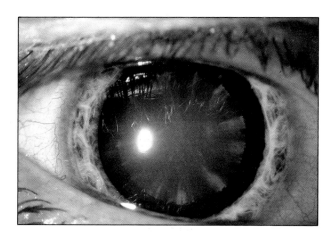

Figure 9.4
Lamellar cataract; note clear periphery of lens

name because it occupies a zone or layer within the lens, indicating that was the embryologically actively developing layer when the lens was subject to some transient insult in utero. About 40 per cent of all congenital cataracts are lamellar (Fig. 9.4).

- **Anterior and posterior polar cataracts**. These lens opacities are confined to the anterior or posterior poles of the lens respectively. Usually they are non-progressive and small, and affect vision to a degree in proportion to their size. They are often associated with fibrous vascular remnants such as a persistent hyaloid artery in the vitreous (Fig. 9.5). In general anterior polar cataracts are much less visually significant than posterior polar cataracts which tend to interfere with vision because they lie close to the optical point in the eye where light rays cross (nodal point).

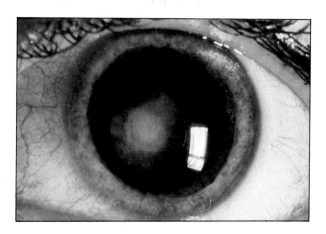

Figure 9.5
Posterior polar congenital cataract

Treatment

Where the cataract is not interfering significantly with the infant's general development and the vision can be assessed as reasonable then no treatment is required. When the infant's vision is severely impaired, as when nystagmus is present, then surgery is required to remove the cataract. For cataracts in the central portion of the lens only, e.g. lamellar or polar cataracts, mydriatic eye drops may be used to keep the pupils dilated which allows adequate vision through the clear lens periphery.

In children with dense bilateral cataracts it is essential to perform surgery at a very early age so that the visual cortex gets some stimulation during its **sensitive period** of development. Delay in undertaking surgery may be associated with cortical visual loss even if the ocular media are made clear. Bilateral cases usually have surgery performed to the second eye very shortly after the first to reduce the risk of amblyopia.

There is much controversy surrounding the treatment of unilateral congenital cataract, as even with surgery these eyes frequently become densely amblyopic unless they have intensive ophthalmic input and patching of the good eye often for many years. There is no doubt that an eye with unilateral congenital cataract can develop good vision with appropriate treatment but it requires a high level of specialist intervention and parent motivation for success. Under these circumstances parents require sensitive counselling as to the advisability of undertaking surgery.

When surgery is required the 'soft' congenital cataract is usually removed by aspiration and/or cutting micro-surgical techniques (lensectomy; Fig. 9.6). After operation patients are rendered aphakic and the high hypermetropic refractive error is usually corrected with contact lenses and/or spectacles both of which are generally tolerated well in small infants. These patients need to be closely monitored for the development of amblyopia and treated appropriately. Intraocular lens implants are generally not used before 2 years of age as the eye is still growing but may be used if surgery is performed after this age or as a secondary procedure when the child is older.

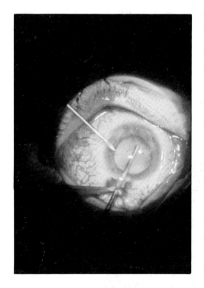

Figure 9.6
'Lensectomy' for congenital cataract

SENILE CATARACT

This type of cataract refers to primary age-associated lens opacities. Senile cataracts form the great majority of all cataracts and can be widely observed in the general population. Almost all people over the age of 65 years have some degree of cataract. They may occur earlier in life (sometimes called pre-senile cataracts) especially in people where nutrition has been poor or who have diabetes mellitus. It is important to distinguish the three types of senile cataract because each type has a different outlook and speed of development. In general however the symptoms of all types of senile cataract are similar.

Symptoms

- Slowly progressive, painless decrease in visual acuity. This may take place over several months or years and usually affects both eyes
- Glare in bright lights and sunlight
- Fixed, dark 'spots' in the field of vision
- Poor colour vision
- Double or multiple images seen with one eye (polyopia).

Types of senile cataract

- **Nuclear sclerosis**. This is a very slow, progressive yellowing and hardening of the lens nucleus. In this way the refractive index of the lens is increased and this renders the patient more myopic (index myopia). In the early stages

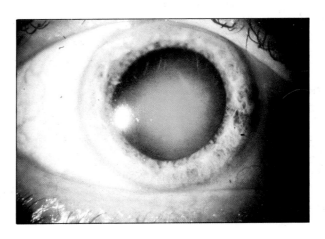

Figure 9.7
Nuclear sclerosis

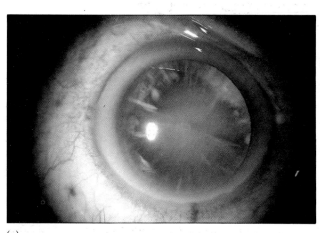

(a)

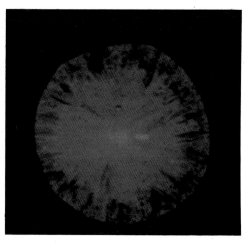

(b)

Figure 9.8 a and b
Cuneiform cataract (a) by direct illumination and (b) seen against the red fundus reflex

such patients continue to see small print and may even be able to abandon their spectacles for reading ('second sight of the aged'). With this type of cataract it is safe to indicate to patients that they will be able to manage to see small print for many years to come even if the distance vision does become progressively blurred (Fig. 9.7).

- **Cortical (cuneiform) cataract.** These are radially arranged spoke-like opacities appearing at the lens periphery both in the anterior and the posterior cortex which slowly extend to the central area of the lens and thereby affect vision. Cortical opacities progress very slowly over many years and patients may be reassured that their progressive visual deterioration will be correspondingly slow (Figs 9.8 a and b).

- **Posterior subcapsular (cupuliform) cataract.** This is another form of cortical cataract but unlike the other two types of senile cataract the opacities progress fairly rapidly. The opacities commence in the central (axial) portion of the lens immediately beneath the posterior lens capsule and extend peripherally. Because of their axial position and because they are close to the optical point of the eye where light rays cross (nodal point), they may have a rapid and profound effect on vision. Patients with this type of cataract generally require surgical intervention soon after presentation (Figs 9.9 a and b).

Nuclear sclerosis, cortical and posterior subcapsular opacities may also occur together or in any combination (e.g.

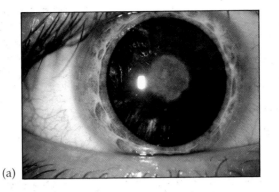

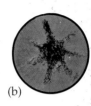

(b)

(a)

Figure 9.9 a and b
Posterior subcapsular cataract (a)
in direct illumination and (b)
against the red fundus reflex

nuclear sclerosis and posterior subcapsular). Nuclear sclerosis occurs particularly in myopic patients, and posterior subcapsular cataract may be associated with systemic steroid treatment.

When a senile cataract occupies the whole lens it is often called a mature cataract and in these circumstances there is no view of the red fundus reflex with the ophthalmoscope and there is a 'white pupil' (Fig. 9.10).

Treatment

Extracapsular cataract extraction and posterior chamber intraocular lens implantation is now the standard technique for cataract surgery and is performed with the operating microscope (Fig. 9.11). This technique requires an incision to

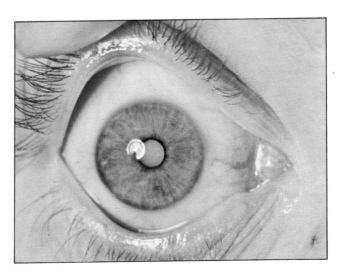

Figure 9.10
Mature or complete cataract

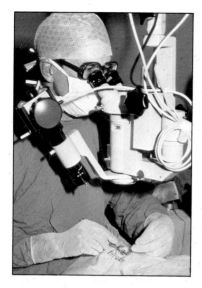

Figure 9.11
General operation view showing
operating microscope

be made in the eye at the corneoscleral limbus (usually in peripheral cornea) through which the lens substance (nucleus and cortex) is removed via a hole (capsulotomy) fashioned in the anterior lens capsule leaving the remaining anterior and posterior lens capsule intact. The remaining 'capsular bag' is used to support the posterior chamber lens implant. Cataract extraction that does not disrupt the posterior lens capsule is highly advantageous as this prevents vitreous humour from passing into the anterior segment of the eye which may be associated with postoperative complications. During traditional extracapsular cataract surgery the nucleus of the lens is then gently expressed from the eye piecemeal through the opening in the anterior capsule and through an incision at the corneoscleral limbus. This approach requires a large (>10 mm) incision to be made in the eye which requires suturing to restore the integrity of the globe. Such sutures may cause corneal astigmatism and consequently affect vision. A more recent method of extracapsular cataract extraction, known as **phacoemulsification**, uses an ultrasonic probe to emulsify and aspirate the lens nucleus whilst it remains in situ (Fig. 9.12). The main advantage of this technique is that it allows a much smaller incision to be made in the eye (4–5 mm) which often does not need suturing and causes less postoperative astigmatism. Phacoemulsification is rapidly becoming the technique of choice for standard cataract surgery. Most patients now have this operation performed as day surgery under local or general anaesthetic. The suitability of the patient for local anaesthetic is determined by factors such as the patient's general health,

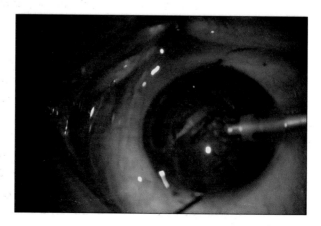

Figure 9.12
Phacoemulsification of
cataractous lens

age and the personal wishes of the patient and the preference of the operating surgeon.

Intracapsular cataract extraction is a technique now seldom used. This operation requires the removal of the lens intact with its capsule by forceps or cryoprobe through a corneoscleral incision. The technique is outdated because it is associated with a higher incidence of complications.

Aphakic vision and intraocular lens implants

Removing a cataractous lens in a patient results in aphakia (absence of the lens). The aphakic eye has lost its power of accommodation and is on average rendered 10 dioptres hypermetropic (long-sighted). In order to see clearly a patient therefore requires the equivalent high-powered convex spectacles, a contact lens or (now routinely used) an intra-ocular lens implant.

Spectacles to correct aphakia have the disadvantage of making the patient entirely dependent on them and require many months of adaptation to the 25% magnified image and peripheral distortion of the spectacle lenses. Judgement of distances especially when pouring liquids and descending steps, is a particular problem.

A contact lens fitted after operation overcomes the high magnification and distortion of spectacles. However, many elderly patients have difficulty in handling a contact lens and regular follow-up examinations may be required.

Intraocular lens (IOL) implants (lens implants) are routinely used because they overcome the disadvantages of spectacles and contact lenses. These implants are traditionally made of polymethylmethacrylate (PMMA) and are inserted into the eye at the time of cataract extraction. The routinely used lens implant is the posterior chamber implant (Fig. 9.13) which is situated exactly in the anatomical position of the original crystalline lens. An extracapsular cataract removal technique is essential for this lens implant to maintain its position.

The introduction of newer materials has led to the development of folding posterior chamber lens implants. These newer lenses are increasingly being used and have the obvious advantage of allowing a smaller corneal incision through which to introduce the folding lens implant. Once

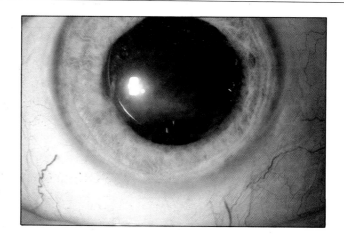

Figure 9.13
Posterior chamber lens implant;
note lower margin of implant not
normally easily seen because it
lies behind the iris

the folding lens is introduced through the small incision it opens up in the capsular bag.

Anterior chamber implants are occasionally used after intracapsular or complicated extracapsular cataract surgery. They may also be used for secondary implantation of previously aphakic patients who do not have adequate capsular remnants to support a posterior chamber implant. The anterior chamber lens implant is held in position by the attached supports in the angle of the anterior chamber (Fig. 9.14).

CATARACT SECONDARY TO OCULAR DISEASE

Many ocular conditions can cause cataracts, the main ones being:

- Prolonged iritis

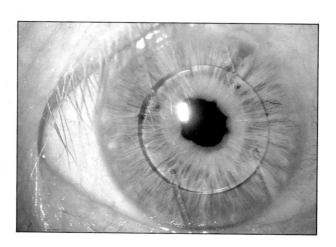

Figure 9.14
Anterior chamber lens implant;
note supporting limbs above and
below

- Injury: both penetrating and non-penetrating injuries, and radiation
- Acute glaucoma
- Retinitis pigmentosa
- Phthisis bulbi: functionally disordered blind eyes, with low intraocular pressure, will almost invariably develop cataract.

CATARACT ASSOCIATED WITH SYSTEMIC DISEASE

A large number of congenital and systemic disorders are associated with cataracts. Some of them are described below:

- **Diabetes mellitus**. The cataracts in diabetes are the same as senile cataracts except that they typically occur a decade or so earlier in diabetics of long standing and progress more rapidly. Diabetics with uncontrolled blood sugar (e.g. undiagnosed) may suffer with variable blurred vision due to osmotic changes within the lens (see Chapter 2).
- **Hypoparathyroidism**. Fine, white, flake-like opacities in the lens cortex, only minimally affecting vision, occur in hypoparathyroidism. The sites of the opacities in the cortex correspond in all probability to the periods of hypocalcaemia.
- **Galactosaemia**. 'Oil droplet', central, congenital cataracts are a frequent feature of this inherited disorder of carbohydrate metabolism. If recognised early the lens changes may be reversible with the exclusion of galactose from the diet.
- **Dystrophia myotonica**. This hereditary disease characterised by frontal baldness, slow relaxation of muscles, generalised muscle wasting giving an expressionless face, and testicular atrophy, is associated with fine, white, dot cataracts sited in the lens cortex.
- **Down's syndrome**. A number of different cataracts occur in this condition which results from a chromosome defect (chromosome 21 trisomy). However, most of these types do not seriously impair vision and seldom require treatment.
- **Systemic steroid treatment**. Patients receiving high-dose systemic steroid therapy over long periods may develop characteristic posterior subcapsular cataracts as a complication.

Displacement of the lens (ectopia lentis)

Complete displacement (dislocation) or partial displacement (subluxation) of the lens may be congenital or acquired. When congenital it is usually symmetrically bilateral and may occur as an isolated anomaly or can be part of a systemic abnormality. Defective suspensory fibres of the zonule holding the lens in place account for the displacement.

Features of a displaced lens

- Tremulousness or 'wobbling' of the iris is apparent (iridodonesis) owing to the iris no longer being supported by the lens.
- Through the dilated pupil the fundus may be observed partly through the lens and partly past the edge of the lens (Fig. 9.15).
- The edge of the displaced lens can often be observed in the pupil.
- The lens may displace into the anterior chamber (anterior dislocation) which may cause secondary glaucoma due to interruption of normal aqueous outflow. When the lens is displaced posteriorly into the vitreous (posterior dislocation) possible complications are cataract, uveitis and secondary glaucoma.
- Rapid changes in the patient's vision associated with rapid changes in refractive error frequently occur with subluxated lenses because of the mobility of the lens. Increasing myopia occurs as the lens moves posteriorly.

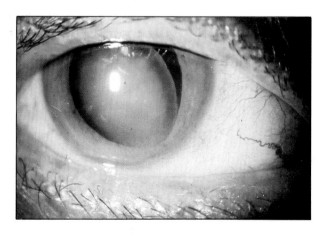

Figure 9.15
Lens subluxation

When the lens is displaced away from the central pupil area the eye is effectively rendered 'aphakic'; the patient therefore requires appropriate spectacles or contact lenses.

- Poor vision is often due to refractive error induced by a displaced lens that is not correctable by spectacles or contact lenses.

Conditions associated with subluxated lenses

- **Marfan's syndrome**. This connective tissue disorder is caused by a mutation in the fibrillin gene. Clinically affected patients have long fingers and toes (arachnodactyly), tall stature, high arched palate and congenital heart defects. Lens subluxation is commonly seen and other ocular features include high myopia, glaucoma and retinal detachment.
- **Homocystinuria**. A metabolic disorder of infants characterised by mental retardation, fair complexion and hair, spastic gait, chest wall deformities and subluxated lenses.
- **Injuries**. Concussion or penetrating injuries to the eye may cause rupture of part of the lens suspensory fibres with consequent lens displacement (see Chapter 8).
- **Age**. Spontaneous rupture of the lens suspensory fibres may occur in older people, especially associated with advanced cataract and myopia.

Treatment of displaced lenses

Partially subluxed lenses can usually be removed by traditional cataract surgical techniques. For a dislocated or severely subluxed lens a vitreolensectomy is the treatment of choice. This procedure involves the removal of the vitreous and displaced lens from a posterior approach.

10 Glaucoma

Anatomy and physiology

Regulation of ocular pressure depends on the balance between the formation and the outflow of aqueous fluid. The aqueous, which is secreted from the ciliary body, flows from the posterior chamber through the pupil into the anterior chamber. It drains out from the eye through the trabecular meshwork in the angle between the cornea and the iris and into the canal of Schlemm, which is a modified vein (Figs 10.1 and 10.2). A small amount of aqueous exits the eye through the outer coats of the eye (uveoscleral outflow). The drainage angle can be viewed clinically on the slit lamp by using a modified contact lens (gonioscope) placed on the anaesthetised cornea (Figs 10.3, 10.4 and 10.5). The normal drainage angle is easily viewed with the gonioscope when it

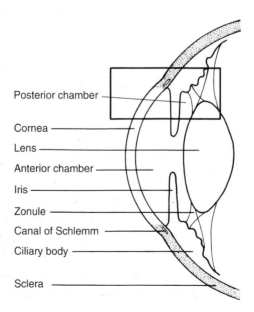

Posterior chamber

Cornea

Lens

Anterior chamber

Iris

Zonule

Canal of Schlemm

Ciliary body

Sclera

Figure 10.1
Anterior segment of the eye

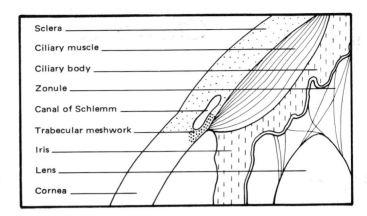

Figure 10.2
The angle of the anterior chamber

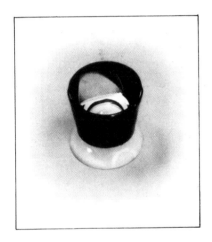

Figure 10.3
The gonioscope

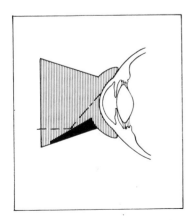

Figure 10.4
The principle of gonioscopy

is described as 'open'. In certain individuals the peripheral iris obscures part or all of the drainage angle, which is then described as 'narrow' or 'closed'. These differences in angle appearance are the basis for classification of different glaucoma types. The constant balance between production of aqueous and its drainage out of the eye maintains the intraocular pressure. The normal range of intraocular pressure is between 9 and 21 mmHg, with an average of 15 mmHg (±3 mm). A rise in intraocular pressure is not caused by increased aqueous secretion but by increased resistance to aqueous outflow from the eye. In acute glaucoma the obstruction to outflow occurs at the periphery of the iris and the intraocular pressure rises rapidly in a short space of time. In chronic glaucoma the site of obstruction is in the trabecular meshwork which causes the pressure to rise over months and even years.

Uncontrolled raised intraocular pressure in glaucoma causes the death of ganglion cell axons. These axons exit the eye in the optic nerve and, as a group, form the neuroretinal rim of the optic disc. The central area of the optic disc is devoid of axons (the optic cup). As glaucomatous damage progresses the amount of axons contributing to the neuroretinal rim reduces. This change is apparent clinically as an increase in the size of the optic cup (**optic disc cupping**; Figs 10.6 and 10.7). In glaucoma ganglion cells supplying the peripheral visual field are damaged first, causing peripheral visual field defects identifiable on field testing but often asymptomatic to the patient. With time the amount of field damage increases so that only a small central island of vision

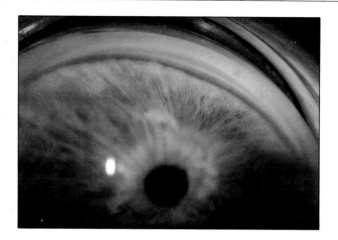

Figure 10.5
Gonioscope view of normal open
angle

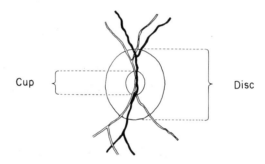

Figure 10.6
The cup/disc ratio

remains (tunnel vision). This central island of vision is usually the last to be affected in glaucoma.

Definition

The word glaucoma is derived from the Greek 'glaucos' meaning green, possibly as a result of an erroneous observation of cataracts in ancient Greece.

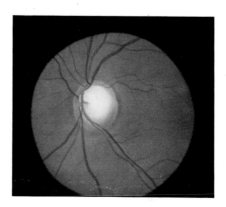

Figure 10.7
A glaucomatous disc showing
excavation (pathological
cupping) and atrophy with a
C/D ratio of 0.8

Glaucoma is a condition usually affecting both eyes in which there is visual field loss, raised intraocular pressure and excavation or pathological cupping of the optic disc. The raised intraocular pressure causes ischaemia of the optic nerve head with ganglion cell death and consequent damage to the retinal nerve fibres, resulting in loss of visual field.

Incidence

The glaucomas are amongst the most important eye diseases in terms of their morbidity and prevalence, accounting for some 5.2 million cases of blindness worldwide. In the developed world 2 per cent of the population over 50 have primary open angle glaucoma rising with age to 4 per cent of the over 80-year-olds. If left untreated glaucoma progresses and leads to irreversible blindness. It accounts for 15 per cent of patients registered as blind.

OCULAR HYPERTENSION

This term is used when the intraocular pressure is above normal but there is no glaucomatous field loss or optic nerve head damage. Elevated intraocular pressure is one of the risk factors for the development of glaucomatous field damage and about 10 per cent of patients with ocular hypertension will go on to develop glaucoma over a 10-year period. Treatment is only required if significant risk factors such as a strong family history of glaucoma are present, or once the intraocular pressure has reached 30 mmHg or more, at which stage there is not only a risk of glaucomatous damage but of a central retinal vein occlusion. Otherwise the patient is monitored.

Classification of glaucoma

- Open angle glaucoma
- Closed angle glaucoma
- Congenital glaucoma.

Open angle glaucoma

PRIMARY OR CHRONIC OPEN ANGLE GLAUCOMA

Primary or chronic open angle glaucoma produces characteristic optic nerve head cupping and visual field loss. It is usually associated with chronically elevated intraocular pressure but the susceptibility to pressure varies between individuals and in some patients relatively minor elevations of intraocular pressure can produce significant disease. Because of the gradual rise of intraocular pressure in chronic glaucoma symptoms may be very gradual and the condition frequently goes unnoticed in the early stages. The condition is usually bilateral and affects those over 40 but is most common after the age of 60 years. It is frequently inherited and some 10 per cent of first-degree relatives of affected individuals also eventually develop glaucoma. For this reason first-degree relatives of glaucoma sufferers are entitled to receive free routine eye examinations after the age of 40 years.

Symptoms

- Loss of part of the visual field; this may be noticed by patients as 'bumping into things', or they may describe an area of field loss.
- Gradual deterioration of close vision; this is more rapid than the usual presbyopic failure of accommodation in those over 40 and the patient may ascribe this failure in vision to the need for stronger reading spectacles.
- Routine medical and optometric examinations frequently detect glaucoma from the appearance of the optic discs, raised intraocular pressure or the detection of visual field loss.

Signs

- The optic disc is pathologically cupped (excavated) and pale, with the central retinal vessels displaced nasally on the disc surface. Evaluation of the size of the cup is helped by observing the cup in relation to the disc (cup:disc or C:D ratio) in the vertical meridian. A disc with a C:D ratio of 0.5 or less is unlikely to be glaucomatous; if greater than 0.5

however it is increasingly likely to be glaucomatous (Figs 10.6 and 10.7).

- Visual field defects occur which can be plotted by perimetry. They are characteristically the arcuate scotoma, an enlarged blind spot and a nasal step defect (Fig. 10.8).
- Raised intraocular pressure usually in the range of 26–40 mmHg measured by tonometry. Tonometry may only satisfactorily be performed by the specialist, using the slit lamp microscope applanation tonometer.

It should be emphasised that these signs are all 'internal' to the eye and there are no apparent external signs. This is in marked contrast to acute glaucoma where all the signs are external.

Treatment

The aim of treatment is to lower the intraocular pressure to prevent further field deterioration and optic disc cupping. Treatment is monitored by regular measurement of intraocular pressure, visual field analysis and assessment of the optic disc.

There are three main treatment options: medical therapy, laser trabeculoplasty and surgical trabeculectomy.

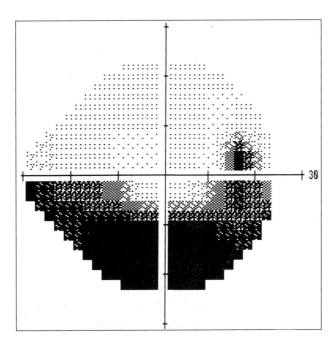

Figure 10.8
Arcuate scotoma in chronic glaucoma

Medical therapy is usually the initial method of treatment, and beta-blockers are generally used as first-line therapy. Combinations of topical therapies are frequently necessary.

- **Beta-blocker eye drops**. Timolol maleate 0.25%–0.5% (Timoptol); betaxolol (Betoptic); carteolol (Teoptic); levobunolol (Betagan) all used twice a day.
  - Action: they work by lowering the production of aqueous humour by inhibiting beta-one and beta-two receptors in the ciliary body. Betoptic has less effect on beta-two receptors.
  - Side effects:
    breathlessness due to bronchospasm (beta-blockers are contraindicated in patients with asthma)
    bradycardia
    reduced exercise tolerance, especially in the elderly.
- **Parasympathomimetic eye drops** (cholinergic eye drops). Pilocarpine 0.5–6% can be used as drops up to four times daily; Pilogel ointment 4% nocte; Ocuserts– these are a soft lens formulation containing pilocarpine, which are inserted weekly and fit in the lower fornix (Fig. 10.9).
  - Action: pilocarpine works by increasing the outflow of aqueous, probably by a mechanical effect with ciliary muscle contraction pulling on and opening the trabecular meshwork.
  - Side effects:
    small pupil
    headache

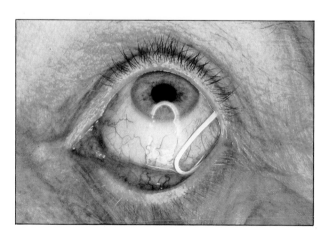

Figure 10.9
Ocusert in position on its way
under upper eyelid

induced myopia

worsening of symptoms of cataract.

- **Sympathomimetic eye drops**. Neutral adrenaline 1% (Eppy); Propine (pro-drug of adrenaline). Both used daily. These preparations are not now commonly used. The success rate of glaucoma surgery is reduced if the patient has been on long-term sympathomimetic therapy prior to surgery.
  - Action: decrease aqueous humour formation.
  - Side effects:
    red eye
    follicular conjunctivitis
    pigmented deposits in lower conjunctiva.
- **Carbonic anhydrase inhibitors**. Acetazolamide (Diamox) tablets, or used i.v. in acute glaucoma; daranide is a similar oral agent; dorzolamide (Trusopt) is a topical carbonic anhydrase inhibitor with few systemic side effects, although patients may complain of a metallic taste and stinging on instillation.
  - Action: decrease aqueous humour production by inhibiting carbonic anhydrase in the ciliary body.
  - Side effects (systemic therapy):
    depression
    malaise
    hypokalaemia
    skin rashes
    poor appetite and gastrointestinal upset
    blood dyscrasias.
- **Alpha-two agonist eye drops**. Brimonidine (Alphagan) used twice daily.
  - Action: reduce aqueous secretion by the ciliary body and increase uveoscleral outflow.
  - Side effects:
    relatively contraindicated in patients with vascular disease
    dry mouth
    fatigue.
- **Prostoglandin F2 alpha agonist eye drops**. Latanoprost (Xalatan), used once a day at night.
  - Action: increases uveoscleral aqueous flow.
  - Side effects:
    bitter taste

turns blue/green eyes brown by increasing melanogenesis in iris melanocytes.

Laser trabeculoplasty is a procedure whereby argon laser burns are placed in the trabecular meshwork to improve aqueous drainage. It has a relatively short duration of action, with a failure rate of 10 per cent per year, and is therefore usually inappropriate for younger patients. It is often beneficial in elderly patients with mild glaucoma or for patients who find difficulty in instilling drops (such as those with arthritis).

Surgical trabeculectomy involves the formation of a surgical fistula from the anterior chamber into the subconjunctival space allowing aqueous to drain out of the eye (Fig. 10.10). If a satisfactory target pressure cannot be reached by medical or laser therapy then trabeculectomy is recommended. Trabeculectomy is able to achieve a greater fall in intraocular pressure than either drugs or laser therapy and is therefore more likely to slow progression of the glaucomatous disease process. Complications of trabeculectomy include reduction in visual acuity, advancement of cataract and occasionally devastating ocular infection (endophthalmitis).

SECONDARY OPEN ANGLE GLAUCOMA

Secondary open angle glaucoma describes features similar to those described above, but arising secondary to an underlying condition. Treatment is directed at the underlying cause as well as the elevated intraocular pressure.

Important causes of secondary open angle glaucoma include the following:

- **Iritis**. Inflammatory cells from the inflamed iris and swelling of angle structures obstruct the outflow of aqueous, causing a rise in intraocular pressure. Treatment of the iritis will settle the problem.
- **Injury**. Injury to the eye may cause damage to the drainage angle obstructing the aqueous outflow. This is called angle recession glaucoma.
- **Steroid eye drops**. Long-term use of steroid eye drops can lead to a secondary rise in intraocular pressure and the

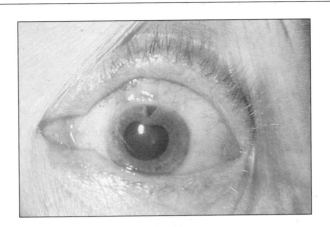

Figure 10.10
Trabeculectomy bleb with
iridectomy

development of glaucoma. For this reason steroid drops
should only be used under close specialist supervision.

- **Pseudoexfoliation**. A curious 'fluffing' of the lens capsule
  called pseudoexfoliation, may cause secondary glaucoma
  (glaucoma capsulare). The areas affected give rise to two
  white ring opacities on the lens capsule. The condition is
  widespread in the population after middle age, is
  discovered mainly on routine examinations, and has an
  especially high incidence in Scandinavia (Fig. 10.11).

Closed angle glaucoma

ACUTE PRIMARY CLOSED ANGLE GLAUCOMA

Acute primary closed angle glaucoma (acute glaucoma)
develops in patients who have an anatomical predisposition
with a narrow anterior chamber drainage angle. It is
particularly prevalent in patients who are highly hypermetropic and have small eyes. The acute attack begins when
the iris and lens become apposed, preventing aqueous in the
posterior chamber from entering the anterior chamber via the
pupil. This **pupil block** tends to occur at night when the pupil
is mid-dilated at which point the gap between the iris and
lens is at a minimum. This causes resistance to aqueous flow
from the posterior to the anterior chamber and pushes the iris
root forwards over the trabecular meshwork. The drainage
angle is then blocked, aqueous cannot drain out of the eye
and the eye pressure rises dramatically. Although normally

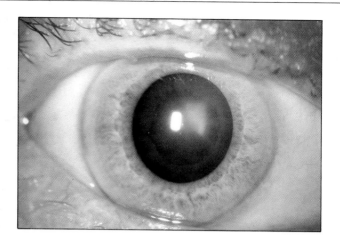

Figure 10.11
Pseudo-exfoliation of lens capsule

only one eye is affected at a time the other eye is at risk of a similar catastrophe. Acute glaucoma develops rapidly over several hours, and produces striking and obvious external eye signs.

Symptoms

- Pain, often severe enough to give rise to nausea and vomiting
- Red, watery, photophobic eye
- Reduced vision due to corneal oedema
- Haloes (rainbow-coloured rings) may be seen around small artificial light sources. This symptom may precede the acute attack, and is due to diffraction in the oedematous cornea.

Signs

- Red eye with dilatation of the ciliary vessels, especially noticeable round the corneal margin (the limbus), giving rise to circumcorneal or ciliary hyperaemia (Figs 10.12 and 10.13)
- Cloudy cornea due to corneal oedema
- Semi-dilated, oval, unreacting pupil
- High intraocular pressure.

Treatment

Acute glaucoma is an ophthalmic emergency; a delay in treatment will inevitably cause damage to the optic nerve

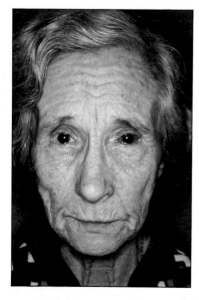

Figure 10.12
Acute glaucoma

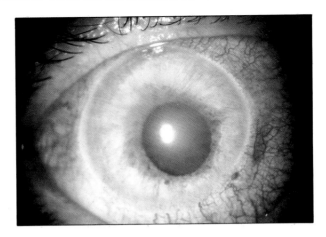

Figure 10.13
The eye signs in acute glaucoma

head and subsequent permanent loss of vision. Treatment involves lowering the intraocular pressure in the affected eye and protecting the uninvolved contralateral eye by prophylactic iridectomy or laser iridotomy. By making an opening between the posterior and anterior chambers the risk of the drainage angle becoming occluded and pupil block developing is removed.

To lower the intraocular pressure oral or intravenous Diamox is given; intravenous mannitol may also be necessary to produce an osmotic diuresis.

Topical beta-blockers and pilocarpine are required and a topical steroid to settle the intraocular inflammation. Once the acute attack has been aborted either a laser iridotomy or a drainage procedure will be required. It must be stressed that because the second eye is at risk of developing acute glaucoma it must be protected by a peripheral iridectomy or laser iridotomy at the same time.

SECONDARY CLOSED ANGLE GLAUCOMA

This unusual form of glaucoma occurs either when the lens and/or iris is pushed forward by some pathology (e.g. choroidal melanoma) causing secondary obstruction of the drainage angle, or when the drainage angle is closed by abnormal tissue (e.g. neovascular glaucoma).

Neovascular (or thrombotic) glaucoma

Secondary glaucoma can develop when the drainage angle is blocked by abnormal new blood vessels. This is usually seen

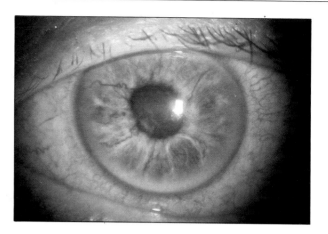

Figure 10.14
Neovascular glaucoma

following ischaemia after a central retinal vein occlusion but may also occur in severe diabetic eye disease. It is extremely difficult to treat and often leads to blindness (Fig. 10.14).

Congenital glaucoma (buphthalmos)

This normally occurs secondary to an abnormal drainage angle formation which may be associated with other ocular abnormalities (Fig. 10.15).

Signs and symptoms

- Photophobia and watering of the eyes
- Enlarged eye or eyes

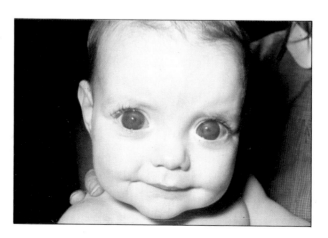

Figure 10.15
Bilateral congenital glaucoma

- Clouding of the corneas
- Poor vision.

If the intraocular pressure is raised in a child less than 2 years old the eye may enlarge. Pathological enlargement after the age of 2 years is unusual.

Treatment

Surgery is the commonest form of management although topical therapy may have to be used in addition or as a holding procedure prior to undertaking operation. Surgery involves making an incision in the abnormal drainage angle or trabeculectomy.

11 Fundus conditions

Anatomy

The normal fundus oculi (when observed with the ophthalmoscope) varies a little between individuals in the background colour (due to variations in retinal pigment) but the optic disc and vessels are remarkably uniform.

The background reddish-orange colour of the fundus is due to the retinal pigment epithelial layer overlying the choroid. Sparse pigmentation (for example in myopia) will allow choroidal vessels to be seen in the fundus. Heavy pigmentation, seen in Asian and African races, gives a deep reddish-orange colour and also a tigroid appearance (likened to a tiger's stripes!). The retina itself is transparent hence the background reddish-orange colour of the pigment epithelial layer and choroid is observed through the retina (Figs 11.1 and 11.2).

The optic disc is the prominent feature of the fundus situated just nasal to the central area of the fundus (the macula). It is slightly oval in shape and marks the commencement of the optic nerve. Fine capillaries cover its surface giving it a lighter red colour in contrast to the darker

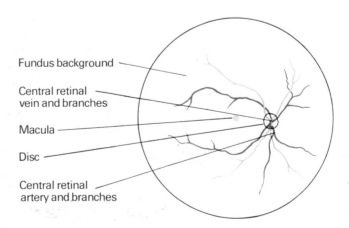

Fundus background

Central retinal vein and branches

Macula

Disc

Central retinal artery and branches

Figure 11.1
The fundus

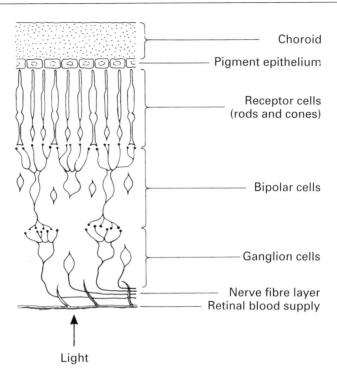

Choroid

Pigment epithelium

Receptor cells
(rods and cones)

Bipolar cells

Ganglion cells

Nerve fibre layer
Retinal blood supply

Light

Figure 11.2
Histological section through the
retina

fundus colour. The disc has clear margins and in its centre a depression called the physiological cup (Figs 11.3 and 11.4).

The retinal blood vessels are observable directly with the ophthalmoscope, the only site in the body where blood vessels can be directly viewed. The veins (or more accurately venules) are observed as columns of bluish blood in transparent vessel walls carrying deoxygenated blood to the central retinal vein at the disc. The arteries (more accurately

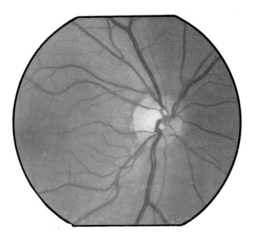

Figure 11.3
The normal fundus

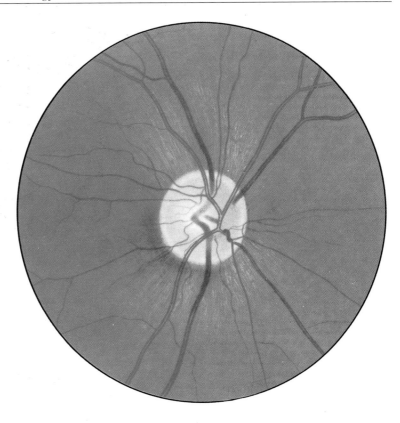

Figure 11.4
The normal fundus: painting

arterioles) are narrower than the veins and appear as red columns of blood in transparent walls carrying oxygenated blood from the central retinal artery away from the optic disc to supply the retina.

The macula is the central feature of the fundus. It appears as a darker red spot on the surrounding fundus with a bright centre point which is the reflected ophthalmoscope light from the minute pit marking the fovea (Fig. 11.5).

Fluorescein angiography of the retina

This technique allows a detailed recorded examination of retinal vascular structure. It is performed by injecting 5 ml of 10% fluorescein solution into the antecubital vein of the patient and then taking a series of monochrome photographs of the fundus in rapid succession about every second. This records the flow of fluorescein through the retinal circulation as it passes in succession through arterioles, capillaries and venules. It demonstrates more clearly than normal ophthal-

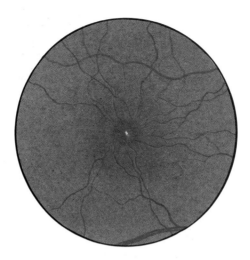

Figure 11.5
The macular region of the normal fundus

moscopy details such as vascular occlusions, leaking abnormal capillaries, microaneurysms and retinal oedema.

Fluorescein angiography is especially valuable in diabetic retinopathy, other retinal vascular disease and choroidal neoplasms (Figs 11.6 and 11.7).

The following fundus conditions will be described:

- Congenital fundus anomalies
- Retinovascular disease
- Senile changes
- Retinal detachment

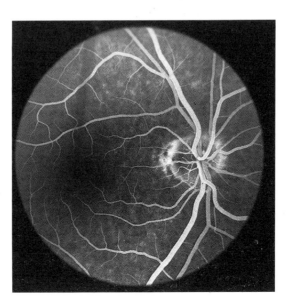

Figure 11.6
Normal fluorescein angiography (late venous phase) showing normal pattern of vessels

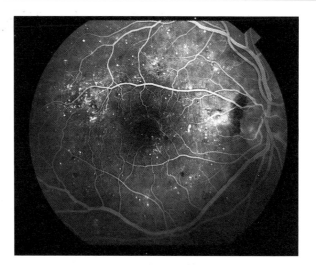

Figure 11.7
Diabetic fluorescein angiography
demonstrating microaneurysms
as brightly fluorescing spots

- Fundus inflammation
- Fundus neoplasms
- Retinal dystrophies.

The fundus abnormalities encountered in diabetes mellitus, hypertension, anaemia and AIDS are covered in Chapter 15.

Congenital fundus anomalies

OPAQUE RETINAL NERVE FIBRES

Retinal nerve fibres are normally non-myelinated but occasionally the myelin sheaths of the optic nerve fibres extend on to the retina as a congenital anomaly. This is seen as a bright white patch adjacent to the disc often obscuring the retinal vessels running in the white patch. Its importance lies in recognising the appearance as a harmless anomaly and it is invariably initially noticed on routine examination of the fundus (Fig. 11.8).

MYOPIC CRESCENT

In congenital and acquired myopia a crescent of white with black pigmented borders may be observed next to the disc.

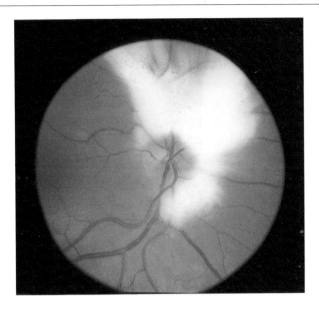

Figure 11.8
Myelinated retinal nerve fibres

The crescent is usually temporal to the disc but may completely surround it. In pathological myopia the myopic crescent will be associated with myopic choroidoretinal degeneration. This crescent is a rim of atrophic choroid revealing the underlying white sclera in a crescent shape (Fig. 11.9).

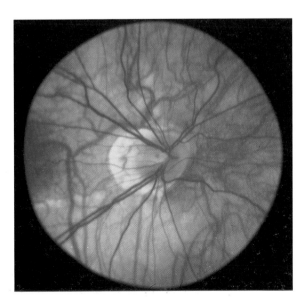

Figure 11.9
Myopic crescent: note prominent choroidal vessels often seen in myopia. (Courtesy of Western Ophthalmic Hospital)

Retinovascular disease

ARTERIOSCLEROSIS

The changes associated with arteriosclerosis of retinal blood vessels must be regarded as normal and are universally seen in the fundi of old people. It is important to recognise these appearances in order to distinguish them from the fundus changes of hypertension (see Chapter 17). They carry no visual symptoms for the patient. Slight narrowing of the retinal arteries giving a brighter reflection of light from the artery surface (the vessel light reflex or reflection), and an irregular calibre of the arterial walls are the principal fundus signs. Nipping of the arteriovenous crossing may also be seen near the disc (Fig. 11.10).

CENTRAL RETINAL ARTERY OCCLUSION

Sudden loss of vision in the affected eye occurs with central artery occlusion and is profound, often with perception of light only remaining. It is in effect infarction of the inner two-thirds of the retina (nerve fibre layer, ganglion and bipolar cells). Recovery is very rare as the central retinal artery is an end artery to the retina which itself is part of the central nervous system. Central retinal artery occlusion usually occurs as a result of thrombosis or embolisation. Less

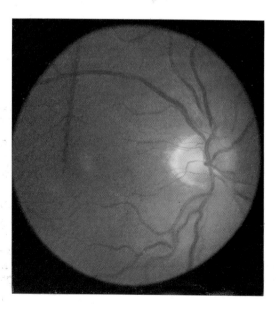

Figure 11.10
Arteriosclerosis of the retinal vessels

common causes include giant-cell arteritis, sickle cell disease and retrobulbar haemorrhage.

The signs are a reduced or absent direct pupil light reflex and the characteristic fundus appearance. A few hours after the event the central fundus looks slightly paler than normal (due to ischaemic retinal swelling obscuring the normal reddish-orange background choroid colour). As the retina is relatively thin in the macular region ischaemic swelling is less marked and the macula looks relatively bright red in contrast to adjacent retina (the 'cherry red' spot) (Fig. 11.11). The retinal arteries are very narrowed. These fundus signs subside over 6–8 weeks to be replaced by a normal fundus background but a very pale disc (optic atrophy).

A **branch retinal artery occlusion** will produce the same fundus signs but confined to the quadrant of supply of the particular branch artery (Fig. 11.12).

Treatment

As the central retinal artery is an end artery its occlusion will rapidly lead to irreversible retinal damage. Complete obstruction of the central retinal artery will cause irreversible retinal damage after around 90 minutes. However as many central retinal artery occlusions are not complete it is possible to get some visual recovery if an embolus can be dislodged within 24 hours. It is essential therefore that patients suspected of suffering a central or branch retinal artery occlusion be assessed by an ophthalmologist as an emergency. Methods employed to dislodge an embolus involve promoting retinal vasculature dilatation (rebreathing exhaled air rich in carbon

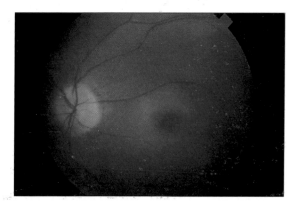

Figure 11.11
Central retinal artery occlusion: note cherry red spot (Courtesy of Western Ophthalmic Hospital)

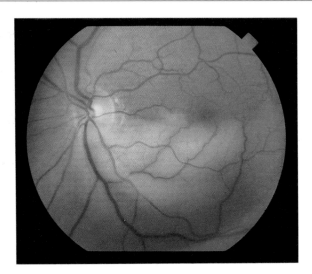

Figure 11.12
Inferior branch retinal artery
occlusion

dioxide) and promoting a precipitous drop in intraocular pressure (ocular massage; systemic acetazolamide; anterior chamber paracentesis). It is important to realise that most central retinal artery occlusions are caused by thrombosis within the central retinal artery and therefore any attempts to dislodge a presumed embolus are often doomed to failure.

CENTRAL RETINAL VEIN OCCLUSION

Sudden loss of vision in the affected eye occurs with central retinal vein occlusion (CRVO) and is usually to a level of 6/60 or less. In some cases visual improvement may occur over several months (in contrast to central retinal artery occlusion). Thrombosis is the usual cause of the occlusion although the exact pathogenesis is not fully understood. Underlying predisposing factors include raised intraocular pressure, hypertension, diabetes mellitus and blood dyscrasias associated with hypercoagulability.

The signs are reduced direct pupil light reflex and characteristic fundus signs. The fundus signs are marked dilatation and tortuosity of the retinal veins, flame haemorrhages over the whole fundus extending to the periphery, cotton-wool spots, macular oedema and swelling of the optic disc (Fig. 11.13). Over several months the signs will gradually disappear and some improvement in vision may occur. Permanent residual fundal signs are sheathing of

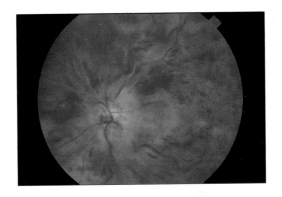

Figure 11.13
Central retinal vein occlusion
(Courtesy of Western Ophthalmic
Hospital)

venules and abnormal tortuous vessel loops (collateral vessels) usually on the optic disc.

Neovascular glaucoma may appear approximately 3 months after a central retinal vein occlusion as a severe and intractable complication.

A **branch retinal vein occlusion** will produce the same fundus signs but confined to the quadrant of the fundus corresponding to the occluded vein (Fig. 11.14). Vision is only affected if the macula is involved and visual reduction is usually less severe than that seen with CRVO. It may also be complicated by neovascularisation, which tends to occur on the optic disc or retina at the junction of ischaemia and non-ischaemic retina and may lead to vitreous haemorrhage.

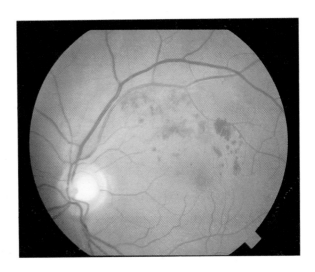

Figure 11.14
Superior branch retinal vein
occlusion

Treatment

Treatment of central retinal or branch vein occlusion should be directed at any underlying cause, e.g. hypertension. Panretinal laser photocoagulation is effective in reversing neovascularisation. Some patients particularly those with branch retinal vein occlusion and chronic macular oedema may benefit from focal macular laser photocoagulation.

Senile changes

AGE-RELATED MACULAR DEGENERATION

As the name implies age-related or senile macular degeneration is largely confined to the elderly and is the most common cause of registrable blindness in Western countries. Patients generally complain of bilateral gradual deterioration of central vision over several years although it may present as sudden deterioration, often with symptoms of distortion.

Frequently the earliest manifestation is small yellow spots called *drusen*, or colloid bodies, scattered round the macular region often associated with pigment speckling. Drusen consist of focal collections of hyaline material between the retinal pigment epithelium and Bruch's membrane. With advancing age they increase in size and number. They are usually an incidental finding and cause no visual symptoms although their presence indicates that the patient is at risk of developing visually significant changes (Fig. 11.15).

- **Non-exudative ('dry' or atrophic) age-related macular degeneration** is characterised by a bilateral progressive atrophy of the retinal pigment epithelium and the choriocapillaries in the macular region secondary to arteriosclerotic degeneration of choroidal vessels. It typically causes a gradual mild to moderate loss of vision over many months or years. Early dry macular degeneration appears as speckled pigmentation followed by the appearance of circumscribed areas of retinal atrophy which allows the underlying larger choroidal vessels to be visualised within the atrophic area (Fig. 11.16). Aside from the provision of low visual aids there is no effective treatment.
- **Exudative age-related macular degeneration** is less

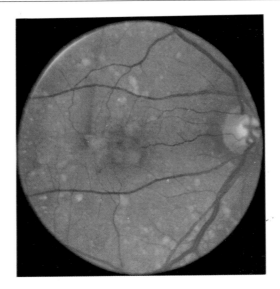

Figure 11.15
Drusen (colloid bodies of the fundus)

common than the dry variety. It causes much more severe visual loss, which may occur rapidly. Patients may present in the early stages with **distortion** of central vision due to retinal oedema or elevation of the retina. The two important features are detachment of the retinal pigment epithelium and choroidal neovascularisation. Choroidal neovascularisation may haemorrhage causing marked visual loss. Organisation following such a haemorrhagic episode leads to the formation of a fibrous **disciform** scar at the macula (Fig. 11.18).

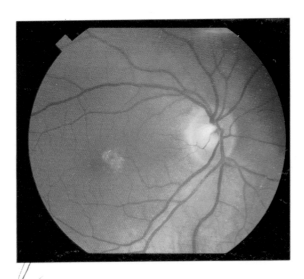

Figure 11.16
Age-related macular degeneration

Treatment

In selected cases argon laser photocoagulation may be effective at destroying a choroidal neovascular membrane. For this reason patients complaining of sudden reduction in central vision particularly if associated with distortion (straight lines appearing bent), should see an ophthalmologist urgently as a small proportion may benefit from laser treatment.

MACULAR HOLE

This degenerative condition generally affects middle-aged women who develop sudden reduction in central vision to around the 6/60 level. Ophthalmoscopically there is a small round retinal hole centred on the fovea (Fig. 11.17). Aetiologically it is thought to be related to vitreous traction acting on the fovea. Treatment with vitrectomy to relieve the tractional forces may cause the hole to close with an improvement in vision.

MYOPIC DEGENERATION

Highly myopic patients tend to have large eyeballs and all retinal layers may be stretched and thinned. Such pathology may lead to a primary choroidal atrophy (Fig. 11.9) which may affect the macular region, or breaks in Bruch's membrane (lacquer cracks) through which choroidal neovascularisation and subsequent disciform scarring may develop in a similar manner to age-related macular degeneration.

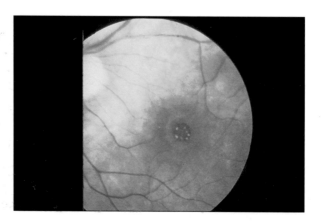

Figure 11.17
Macular hole

ANGIOID STREAKS

As their name implies angioid streaks have an ophthalmoscopic appearance similar to blood vessels. They are irregular, reddish streaks that extend outwards from the optic disc and are usually asymptomatic unless they affect the macular region. They represent cracks in Bruch's membrane through which choroidal neovascularisation and disciform scarring may occur (Fig. 11.18). Angioid streaks may be associated with pseudoxanthoma elasticum, Ehlers–Danlos syndrome, Paget's disease and sickle-cell anaemia.

Retinal detachment

This is a condition in which the retina becomes separated from its pigment epithelial layer. The separation occurs at this site for embryological reasons: the two walls of the embryonic optic vesicle become apposed and form respectively the retinal pigment epithelium and the neuroretina. There are two main types of retinal detachment:

- **Rhegmatogenous retinal detachment**. By far the most common type it occurs secondary to a tear or hole in the retina, which often arises as a consequence of posterior vitreous detachment.
- **Non-rhegmatogenous (exudative and tractional) retinal detachment**. An uncommon type in which retinal detachment occurs without a defect in the retina. It arises either as a result of exudative processes beneath the retina (e.g.

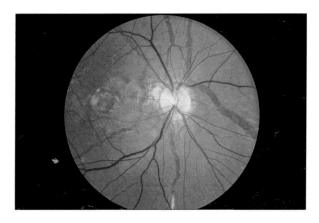

Figure 11.18
Angioid streaks with disciform macular degeneration

scleritis or choroidal neoplasm) or as a result of vitreous tractional forces pulling the retina forward (e.g. proliferative diabetic retinopathy).

The remainder of this section will be concerned with rhegmatogenous retinal detachment only.

Retinal detachment is most common after the age of 50 years and is commonest in patients with high myopia. Trauma plays a part in younger patients. A lower incidence is reported in African races. Certain systemic connective tissue disorders, notably Marfan's and Stickler's syndromes, are associated with an increased risk of retinal detachment.

Symptoms

Sudden onset of floating specks or spots associated with flashes of light in the affected eye are typical symptoms of posterior vitreous detachment and/or retinal tear formation. The same day or days or weeks later a 'shadow' or 'curtain' in the visual field can be seen that gradually extends to cover the whole visual field.

Signs

Reduced visual acuity will be marked if the macular region becomes detached. There will be visual field loss corresponding to the area of detached retina, e.g. the temporal retina generally detaches first thereby giving a nasal field defect. The detached retina may be seen with the ophthalmoscope as a greyish area and as retinal folds which quiver as the eye moves. The blood vessels on the detached part of the retina appear a deeper red colour than normal. If an area of retina still remains in situ an easy contrast between the normal fundus colour and the greyish detached portion can be observed. A retinal break will be seen at the periphery of the detached fundus in the form of a tear ('arrowhead' or 'U' shaped), a hole or a dialysis. The dialysis is particularly associated with trauma (Figs 11.19 and 11.20).

Treatment

A retinal detachment usually requires surgical repair. The principles of this operation are to seal the retinal break by

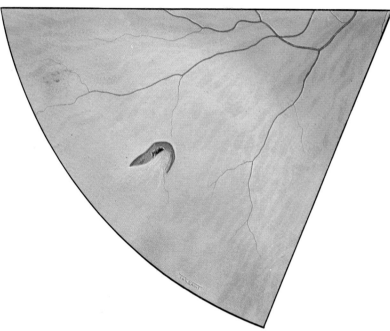

Figure 11.19
U-shaped retinal tear and
detachment

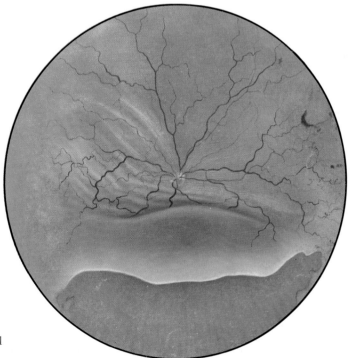

Figure 11.20
Retinal detachment with retinal
dialysis

inducing retinal scarring with laser or cryotherapy and to relieve vitreous traction over the break, either by attaching an indenting implant of silastic to the sclera or by vitrectomy. The visual prognosis depends on the duration of the detachment and whether the macula has been detached.

Asymptomatic retinal tears and holes may sometimes be seen on routine examination of the fundus. Similarly, retinal tears may be found in patients presenting with symptoms of flashes and floaters. Untreated such tears may ultimately lead to retinal detachment which may be prevented by laser photocoagulation or retinal cryotherapy. Prevention of retinal detachment is clearly preferable to surgery and it is therefore important that patients with appropriate symptoms have urgent ophthalmic assessment.

Fundus inflammation

Inflammation of the choroid (choroiditis or posterior uveitis) causes rapid blurring of vision, usually in one eye, with 'spots' and 'haziness' over the whole visual field (due to inflammatory cells in the vitreous). Because the choroid and retina lie next to each other inflammation of the choroid always affects the overlying retina to produce a chorio-retinitis. Cytomegalovirus (CMV) chorioretinitis associated with AIDS is covered in Chapter 15.

TOXOPLASMOSIS

The toxoplasmosis parasite (a protozoan, *Toxoplasma gondii*) probably causes choroiditis by its entry into the bloodstream via ingested infected material from wild or domestic cats. The parasite may be transmitted across the placenta causing congenital toxoplasmosis.

Many people are unaware they have had a toxoplasmosis chorioretinitis in childhood or from birth until a characteristic old fundus lesion is noted on routine examination in later years. Toxoplasmosis primary infection in adults may be accompanied by a mild febrile illness that precedes the eye symptoms.

Signs and symptoms

Active toxoplasmosis chorioretinitis causes reduced vision, a very hazy view of the fundus (because of the inflammatory cells in the vitreous) and a localised white fluffy area in the fundus. If the active episode follows an earlier primary or congenital infection (as is usually the case) the active focus normally arises from an area adjacent to a pigmented chorioretinal scar. If this is the case then the current active episode is recurrent rather than primary. Distinguishing recurrent from primary disease is particularly important in pregnancy, as primary infection poses a risk of congenital toxoplasmosis to the foetus whereas recurrent disease does not. Serological tests for toxoplasma antibodies may be of use in aiding diagnosis and differentiating between primary and recurrent infections. The fundus signs change as the chorioretinitis subsides over many weeks and finally there remains a heavily pigmented, circumscribed area of choroidal atrophy (Figs 11.21 and 11.22).

Treatment

Treatment of toxoplasmosis chorioretinitis depends on visual impairment, or on its potential to cause visual loss. Treatment is usually commenced when there is severe vitritis or the active lesion is close to the macula or optic disc. Peripheral retinal foci of chorioretinitis may be left untreated as they do not threaten central vision and natural resolution may be

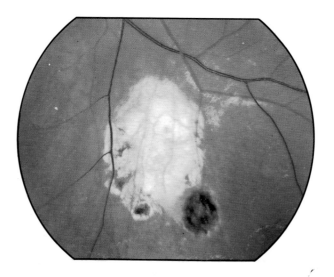

Figure 11.21
Recurrence of choroiditis adjacent to old toxoplasmosis pigmented area of choroido-retinal atrophy

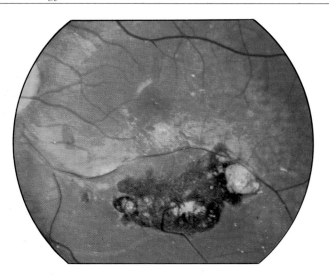

Figure 11.22
Area of old, inactive choroiditis
due to toxoplasmosis

awaited. Oral treatment consists of corticosteroids with a combination of pyrimethamine, sulphadiazine or clindamycin.

TOXOCARIASIS

Eggs from the dog tapeworm, *Toxocara canis*, may be ingested by contact with infected excreta. These eggs hatch in the gut and the larvae migrate throughout the body via the blood and lymphatic system. In children larvae invading the eye may cause a focal chorioretinitis (Fig. 11.23) or an endophthalmitis and leukocoria.

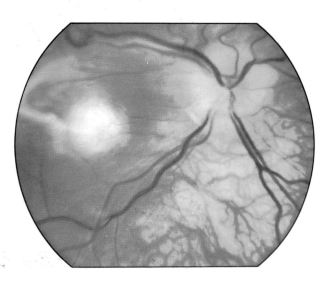

Figure 11.23
Toxocariasis choroiditis

HISTOPLASMOSIS

This is a fungus infection endemic in some parts of North America. The choroiditis caused by this infection produces peripheral small areas of choroiditis but also may produce rapid visual loss because of choroidal neovascularisation, macular haemorrhage and disciform scarring.

Fundus neoplasms

BENIGN MELANOMA OF THE CHOROID

Often called a choroidal naevus, a benign melanoma of the choroid is invariably asymptomatic and discovered only on routine ophthalmoscopic examination.

The ophthalmoscopic appearance is of a localised, flat, even, brown patch on the fundus, often with overlying drusen. As it is within the choroid overlying retinal blood vessels traverse the lesion uninterrupted. Benign melanomata are usually in the posterior pole of the fundus and are about the size of the optic disc. There is no associated visual field defect (Fig. 11.24).

MALIGNANT MELANOMA OF THE CHOROID

This primary malignant tumour of the choroid is most frequent in middle life.

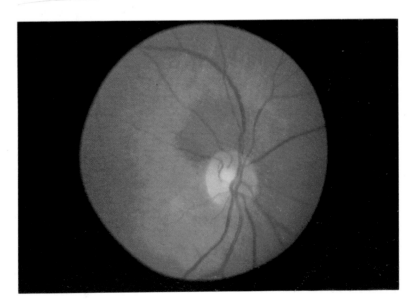

Figure 11.24
Benign choroidal melanoma
adjacent to disc

Symptoms

Symptoms are similar to those of retinal detachment, namely an increasing 'shadow' or 'curtain' in the field of vision over a period of weeks. If a secondary (exudative) retinal detachment occurs involving the macula rapid visual loss will occur over a few days.

The ophthalmoscopic appearance is of a raised brown or grey area near the posterior pole of the fundus often with overlying orange pigmentation. With a large tumour there is frequently an associated exudative retinal detachment. A visual field defect, corresponding to the site of the tumour, is present (Fig. 11.25).

Fluorescein angiography of the fundus, ultrasonography and magnetic resonance imaging (MRI) may aid diagnosis and detect extraocular extension. Malignant melanoma metastasises widely in an unpredictable manner often after many years.

Treatment

Treatment consists of either removal of the affected eye or localised radiotherapy to the eye in the case of small tumours. Occasionally very small tumours may be treated with laser photocoagulation. There is some doubt whether early removal of the eye affects the prognosis for life but clearly,

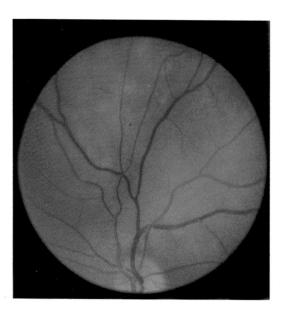

Figure 11.25
Malignant choroidal melanoma superiorly; note the raised vessels and greyish appearance

where vision has been lost in an eye with a malignant melanoma, removal is desirable.

RETINOBLASTOMA

See Chapter 14.

SECONDARY TUMOURS

Primary tumours elsewhere in the body (especially carcinoma of the breast and bronchus) may give rise to secondary choroidal tumours. There is usually clinical evidence of the primary tumour site.

The patient may complain of blurred vision or a 'shadow' in the visual field. The secondary choroidal tumour appears by ophthalmoscopy as a raised greyish-yellow area at the posterior pole of the fundus.

Treatment

Treatment of the secondary tumour in the choroid may occasionally be justified in the form of localised radiotherapy to the eye. However the presence of a secondary choroidal tumour invariably indicates widespread metastases, so death occurs fairly soon after the diagnosis is made.

Retinal dystrophies

RETINITIS PIGMENTOSA (RP)

This condition is an inherited primary retinal degeneration. The mode of inheritance varies between different families as does the severity of the disease. There may be associations with systemic disorders (e.g. Usher's syndrome of RP and congenital sensorineural deafness).

Symptoms

Night blindness in childhood or adolescence is the initial symptom. Following this there is gradual and progressive peripheral visual field loss leading eventually to 'tunnel vision'. The rate of progression varies greatly and in general the later the onset the less severe the final outcome.

Signs

Visual field loss in the early stages is characteristically in the form of a ring scotoma progressing later to total constriction of the visual fields ('tunnel vision'). The fundus appearance shows the classical mid-periphery scattered 'bone spicule' pigmentation, marked narrowing of the retinal vessels and optic atrophy (Fig. 11.26).

At the present time there is no known effective treatment.

MACULAR DYSTROPHIES

Progressive degeneration of the maculae may occur in children and young adults usually as a hereditary disorder. There are several varieties of this disorder (Best's disease, cone dystrophy, pattern dystrophy), all leading to slow deterioration in central vision which may be noticed on routine vision screening in children or in young adults presenting with progressive visual failure.

The signs of this disorder are reduced visual acuity and abnormal deposits or pigmentation ('Bull's eye') at the macula (Fig. 11.27). Electrophysiological testing is often

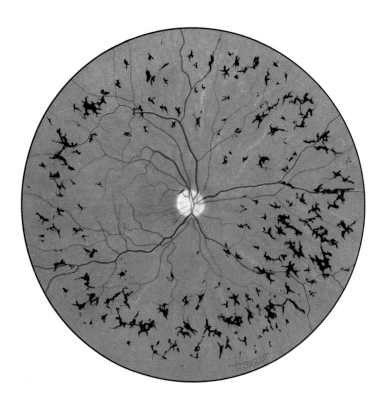

Figure 11.26
Retinitis pigmentosa

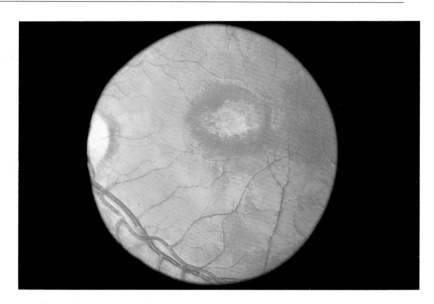

Figure 11.27
Macular dystrophy

useful in establishing a precise diagnosis. No treatment is effective but special low vision aids (e.g. telescopic spectacles) may be of significant visual benefit and allow a normal education.

12 Neuro-ophthalmology

Anatomy

The optic nerve contains approximately 1.2 million axons from the ganglion cell layer of the retina. These axons are unmyelinated as they traverse the retina but gain a myelin sheath as they enter the optic nerve. The axons pass through the optic chiasma (where the axons from the nasal retina decussate) into the optic tract. The axons synapse in the lateral geniculate body from where the next order of neurones arise to form the optic radiation which extends to the visual cortex in the occipital lobe. Posterior to the optic chiasma the visual pathways are arranged such that information from the right visual field passes to the left occipital lobe and information from the left visual field passes to the right occipital lobe (Fig. 12.1).

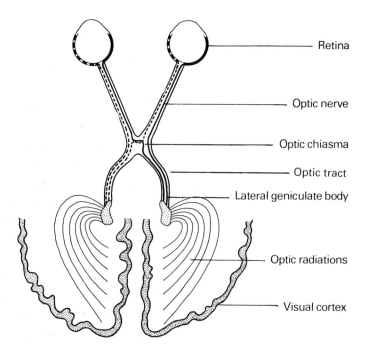

Retina

Optic nerve

Optic chiasma

Optic tract

Lateral geniculate body

Optic radiations

Visual cortex

Figure 12.1
The visual pathway

The parasympathetic nervous supply to the eye arises in the brain stem close to the IIIrd cranial nerve nucleus and travels with the IIIrd cranial nerve to reach the eye, where it supplies the constrictor pupillae muscle of the iris and the ciliary muscle. The sympathetic nervous supply to the eye follows a circuitous route, arising in the hypothalamus descending in the brain stem and spinal cord exiting at the level of the first thoracic vertebra (T1) then ascending to synapse in the superior cervical ganglion and pass to the eye in association with its arterial vascular supply. It innervates the dilator pupillae muscle of the iris and the smooth muscle part of the levator palpebrae superioris muscle.

This chapter will cover the following conditions:

- Optic nerve disease
- Visual pathway disorders
- Cranial nerve palsies
- Other conditions.

Optic nerve disease

Damage to the optic nerve can be seen clinically with the ophthalmoscope in the form of optic disc swelling or pallor (optic atrophy).

OPTIC DISC SWELLING

Swelling of the optic disc is produced by oedema within the nerve head. The causes of optic disc swelling are:

- **Raised intracranial pressure**. Intracranial tumours or impaired CSF drainage cause raised intracranial pressure which is transmitted to the meningeal sheath surrounding the optic nerve. This results in the clinical appearance of optic disc swelling (**papilloedema**) due to interruption of normal axoplasmic flow at the optic nerve head with consequent intra-axonal swelling. The vascular features (hyperaemia, venous congestion and haemorrhage) are all secondary.
- **Ischaemia**. **Ischaemic optic neuropathy** is caused by arteritic, embolic or atherosclerotic blockage of the posterior ciliary arteries which supply the optic nerve head. This produces ischaemia at the optic nerve head with

interruption of axoplasmic flow and disc swelling. Central retinal vein occlusion and malignant hypertension may be associated with a swollen optic disc for similar reasons.

- **Inflammation**. This is called papillitis or optic neuritis. It may be idiopathic or be associated with multiple sclerosis, diabetes or post-viral infection.
- **Compression**. Raised intraorbital pressure (e.g. Graves' disease, retrobulbar haemorrhage) or a tumour may compress the optic nerve causing optic disc swelling.
- **Infiltration**. Occasionally an optic nerve may be subject to an infiltrative process (e.g. lymphoma), causing disc swelling.
- **Toxic**. Steroids, ethambutol and tobacco may cause a toxic optic neuropathy associated with disc swelling or pallor.
- **Trauma**. Direct or indirect trauma to the optic nerve may cause optic disc swelling and subsequent optic atrophy.

The term papilloedema should be restricted to a swollen optic disc due to raised intracranial pressure and it is better to refer to a swollen disc simply as such until the underlying cause is known.

Symptoms

- Impaired vision: vision may be affected to a variable extent depending on the cause of the disc swelling. Raised intracranial pressure may cause no visual symptoms, but is more often associated with transient blurring of vision (visual obscurations). Ischaemia of the disc in giant-cell arteritis, or inflammation of the disc in optic neuritis, may cause very rapid and severe visual loss.
- Visual field loss: raised intracranial pressure may be associated with an enlargement of the blind spot on visual field testing but usually causes no symptomatic field loss. Ischaemic optic neuropathy typically causes an altitudinal visual field defect. Compression and toxicity usually causes a central or centrocaecal visual field defect.
- Impaired colour vision: particularly to red stimuli.
- Pain on eye movements is typical of optic neuritis.

Signs

- Dilatation of the retinal veins

- Reddish disc colour with blurred and raised disc margins (Fig. 12.2)
- Absence of central physiological cup on the disc (filled in by oedema)
- Small haemorrhages at the disc margin
- The pupil light reflex is reduced in certain conditions causing disc swelling
- Enlarged blind spot or other characteristic defects on visual field plotting
- Impaired colour vision.

CONDITIONS CAUSING SWOLLEN DISCS

Intracranial tumours

Tumours in the posterior cranial fossa are particularly liable to cause papilloedema.

Hypertension

Disc swelling will always be accompanied by the other fundus signs of hypertension. When disc swelling is present the term malignant hypertension is sometimes used and implies an acute marked rise in blood pressure (see Chapter 15).

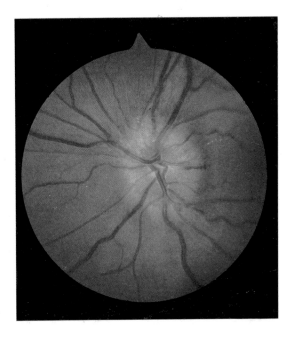

Figure 12.2
Swollen disc (papilloedema)

Central retinal vein occlusion

Sudden loss of vision characterises an occlusion of the central retinal vein and the disc swelling will always be accompanied by the other fundus signs (see Chapter 11).

Giant-cell arteritis (temporal or cranial arteritis)

This condition is largely confined to those over 70 years with sudden loss of vision in one or both eyes. The affected arteries may be any in the head and neck. If the posterior ciliary arteries are affected there is swelling of the optic disc (ischaemic optic neuropathy) and loss of vision. Optic atrophy occurs after some months. Urgent treatment with high-dose corticosteroids is aimed at preventing involvement of the second eye (see Chapter 15).

Multiple sclerosis (MS)

Most common in temperate climates this widespread neurological disease affects young adults mostly between the ages of 15–35 years. Women are more commonly affected than men. The aetiology is unknown; however some evidence suggests the disorder may arise as a result of a slow virus infection of the nervous system. Optic neuritis is the main ophthalmological sign which arises as a result of demyelination of optic nerve axons.

Blurring of vision in one eye occurring over a few days, is the presenting feature of many patients with MS. The visual loss is variable and ranges from minimal loss of vision to perception of light only (usually around 6/60). The scotoma is usually central with preserved peripheral vision. Gradual recovery of vision usually occurs over several weeks. Pain on moving the eye is often present.

Whilst the other signs are constant the disc swelling may not always be observed if the area of optic neuritis occurs well behind the optic disc (**retrobulbar neuritis**). Other signs of multiple sclerosis may be present or follow later such as ataxia, parasthesiae, nystagmus and strabismus. Following an isolated attack of adult optic neuritis the risk of developing MS is approximately 50 per cent. MRI scanning of the central nervous system may show plaques of demyelination in patients who will subsequently develop MS. The diagnosis of optic neuritis can be confirmed by demonstrating delay in conduction of the visually evoked response.

Optic neuritis may occur in children following a postviral infection when it is often bilateral. Optic neuritis occurring in adults is usually either idiopathic or associated with MS, where it is often the presenting complaint.

OPTIC ATROPHY

Any damage to the optic nerve from whatever cause, will result in degeneration of the optic nerve fibres and destruction of their myelin nerve sheaths. The dead nerve fibre axons are replaced by glia which give the atrophic disc its typical ophthalmoscopic pale appearance. Optic atrophy may be primary or secondary.

Primary optic atrophy

Optic atrophy may occur congenitally and often has a hereditary basis.

Secondary optic atrophy

Any cause of optic disc swelling may be followed by the development of optic atrophy (see above). Several of these disorders may cause optic atrophy without an observed episode of disc swelling (e.g. optic nerve compression and toxic optic neuropathy).

Certain retinal disorders do not cause optic disc swelling but do cause optic atrophy. These include glaucoma, retinitis pigmentosa and central retinal artery occlusion.

Signs and symptoms

- Focal or generalised disc pallor (Fig. 12.3)
- The disc margins appear sharper because of the contrast between the pale disc and fundus colour
- Diminished visual acuity
- Visual field loss depending on the precise cause of the optic atrophy.

The history, visual field plotting, other associated signs and appropriate investigations will lead to an accurate assessment of the cause of the optic atrophy.

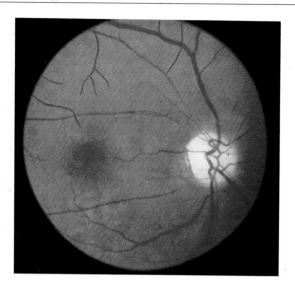

Figure 12.3
Optic atrophy

TOXIC AND NUTRITIONAL OPTIC ATROPHY

This cause of optic atrophy deserves particular mention as it is one of the few causes amenable to treatment. Very slow and progressive visual failure of both eyes with loss of colour vision occurs with poisoning by a number of toxic agents. The visual deterioration takes place over many months and even years.

Agents causing this slowly progressive optic atrophy are quinine and its derivatives (used as antimalarials and for relieving night cramps) and strong tobaccos. Vitamin B deficiencies are also a causative factor. It seems that certain individuals are prone to the toxic effects of tobacco especially when combined with poor nutrition and high alcohol intake (tobacco–alcohol amblyopia).

The signs of toxic and nutritional optic atrophy are diminished visual acuities, characteristic centrocaecal (extending from blind spot to fixation) scotomata and pallor of the optic discs (Fig. 12.4).

Treatment

Treatment consists of withdrawing the toxic agents, replacing any vitamin deficiency and a long-term course of intramuscular injections of hydroxocobalamin (vitamin B12).

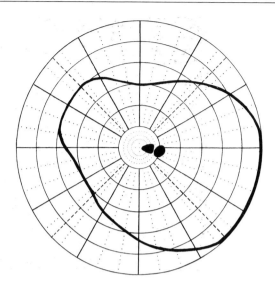

Figure 12.4
Centrocaecal scotoma field defect in toxic optic atrophy

Visual pathway disorders

Disorders of the optic chiasma, optic tract, optic radiations and visual (occipital) cortex manifest themselves as defects in the visual fields.

PITUITARY TUMOURS: CHIASMAL COMPRESSION

Pituitary tumours are slowly expanding lesions (usually chromophobe adenomata) and because the optic chiasma lies immediately above the pituitary gland it is slowly compressed. Other lesions which can cause similar chiasmal compression are craniopharyngioma (mainly in children, arising above chiasma), suprasellar meningioma and carotid aneurysms.

Signs and symptoms

As fibres from the nasal retina of each eye cross in the optic chiasma they will be affected first by any compressive pathology causing the classical **bitemporal hemianopia**.

Chiasmal compression may be asymptomatic in its early stages. More severe or prolonged compression may cause symptoms of 'bumping into things' at the side and slight loss of visual acuity. Other patients may complain of diplopia (due to the difficulty in fusing two complementary half fields) or an inability to see objects behind the object of regard (post-fixational blindness; the bitemporal hemianopic field crosses behind the object of fixation).

The signs are characteristic and consist of bilateral pale discs, reduced visual acuity and bitemporal hemianopia (commencing superotemporally because of the initial compression of the underside of the optic chiasma) (Fig. 12.5). With severe or very prolonged chiasmal compression fibres from the temporal retina will also be damaged and this may ultimately cause extensive visual field defects and blindness.

Investigation and treatment

Skull X-rays may show an expanded pituitary fossa or suprasellar calcification suggestive of craniopharyngioma. CT and MRI scans are more sensitive investigations that can show bony expansion and extent of tumour mass respectively. In patients with a suspected pituitary tumour a full endocrine assessment is mandatory.

Most expanding chromophobe adenomata pituitary tumours require surgical removal to prevent progressive visual loss. The eosinophil adenomata that give rise to the clinical picture of acromegaly and gigantism frequently spare the optic chiasma and their removal is not often required. Basophil adenomata may produce Cushing's disease through secretion of ACTH but they do not expand sufficiently to cause chiasmal compression.

OPTIC TRACT, OPTIC RADIATION AND VISUAL CORTEX CONDITIONS

Any pathology affecting the optic tract, optic radiation or visual (occipital) cortex will cause a contralateral **homonymous hemianopia**; loss of vision in one half of the visual field in each eye (Fig. 12.6). Such pathology is often vascular in origin caused by occlusion of branches of the middle and posterior cerebral arteries. As such homonymous hemianopia is common in patients who have suffered a stroke. Other causes include cerebral tumours, aneurysms and multiple sclerosis. Migraine is commonly associated with a transient homonymous hemianopia.

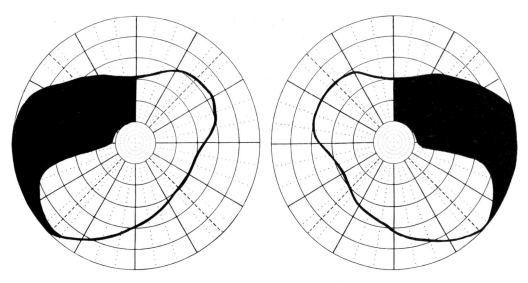

Figure 12.5
Bitemporal hemianopia field
defect in chiasmal compression

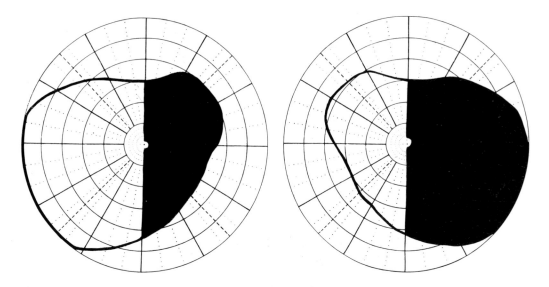

Figure 12.6
Homonymous hemianopia visual
field defect

Signs and symptoms

With vascular lesions behind the optic chiasma patients
notice sudden loss of vision in one half of the visual field in
each eye. They commonly only notice the visual field loss in
the eye with the larger temporal field loss and fail to notice
the similar loss in the nasal field of the other eye. With

cerebral tumours this visual field loss is gradual in onset and slowly progressive. Visual acuity is usually normal as at least half of the macular fibres will be unaffected.

Examination shows normal pupil light reflexes, normal fundi and a homonymous hemianopia. Segmental optic atrophy may be seen in lesions affecting the optic tract only.

Visual field recovery following a vascular homonymous hemianopia is uncommon. Relief of a compressive lesion or resolution of a demyelinating episode may be associated with improvement of visual fields.

Cranial nerve palsies

Cranial nerve palsies may be congenital or acquired. Isolated acquired cranial nerve palsies may arise as a result of localised microvascular disease (particularly with hypertension or diabetes), compression by tumours or aneurysm, demyelination, raised intracranial pressure (especially VIth cranial nerve) or trauma. A brainstem cerebrovascular accident (CVA) is a common cause of cranial nerve palsy and is associated with other neurological deficits.

IIIrd (OCULOMOTOR) NERVE PALSY

IIIrd nerve palsies account for one-third of acquired ocular cranial nerve palsies and may be complete or incomplete. The IIIrd nerve supplies all of the extraocular muscles excluding superior oblique and lateral rectus. Palsy causes the eye to be divergent and hypotropic with a ptosis (Fig. 12.7). The ocular

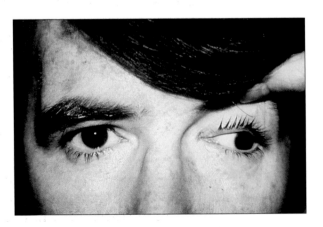

Figure 12.7
Left IIIrd nerve palsy

movements on the affected side are usually extremely poor. The pupil may or may not be involved but a fixed dilated pupil suggests a compressive lesion (most commonly a posterior communicating artery aneurysm) and urgent neurosurgical help and advice is required. Occasionally in these circumstances the pupil fibres will be affected before an ocular motility problem arises. Pain is characteristic in IIIrd palsy caused by aneurysmal compression.

The majority of IIIrd nerve palsies are microvascular in aetiology and spontaneous improvement is common usually within 3 months. If the patient has a complete ptosis, then no double vision is perceived. If however the ptosis is incomplete prisms or patching can be considered to alleviate the situation whilst awaiting spontaneous improvement. If there is no improvement within 12–18 months surgery can be considered but it is often difficult to realign the eyes and attain single vision.

IVth (TROCHLEAR) NERVE PALSY

IVth nerve palsy is the commonest congenital palsy but it accounts for less than 10 per cent of acquired ocular cranial nerve palsies. Acquired palsies tend to follow relatively minor closed head trauma such as occurs in head injuries without loss of consciousness. Bilateral palsies are common following this sort of injury but are often overlooked. The IVth nerve supplies the superior oblique muscle only and palsy therefore causes vertical diplopia which is often worse on downward gaze. The patient will often use a compensatory head tilt to the unaffected side to eliminate the diplopia. In a uniocular IVth nerve palsy the eye is hypotropic and there is a weakness of depression in adduction. Surgery can be extremely helpful in patients with congenital and acquired IVth nerve palsies to reduce the diplopia and/or head tilt. Bilateral palsies are more difficult to treat than unilateral palsies.

VIth (ABDUCENS) NERVE PALSY

VIth nerve palsy accounts for 50 per cent of acquired ocular cranial nerve palsies. The VIth nerve supplies the lateral rectus muscle only and palsy leads to an incomitant convergent strabismus which is most marked when looking

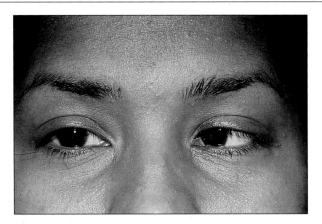

Figure 12.8
Right VIth nerve palsy (note reduced abduction on looking to the right side)

in the direction of action of the palsied muscle (i.e. impaired abduction of the affected eye) (Fig. 12.8). Patients generally complain of double vision which may only be present in the distance. They may demonstrate a compensatory head posture with a face turn to the affected side. These palsies are often of microvascular aetiology and therefore spontaneous recovery of acquired palsies within 3 months is usual. In a patient with a VIth nerve palsy the fundus should always be examined to check for papilloedema as the palsy may be a false localising sign of raised intracranial pressure.

The initial treatment is with a prism or patch to cover the affected eye thereby removing double vision. Treatment is expectant of spontaneous improvement but if recovery has not occurred after 3 months botulinum toxin therapy may be considered to weaken the medial rectus muscle and try to encourage lateral rectus muscle function. If this does not produce a cure surgery can be considered after 12–18 months.

VIIth (FACIAL) NERVE PALSY

Facial nerve palsy is commonly seen following a brainstem CVA, Bell's palsy or trauma. Ocular features arise from denervation of the orbicularis oculi muscle and include brow droop (if lower motor neurone lesion), lagophthalmos (poor eye closure), lower lid ectropion and epiphora (Fig. 12.9). Poor blink and eye closure may lead to corneal exposure keratitis which can usually be prevented by using topical lubricants and taping the eye closed at night. Surgery to

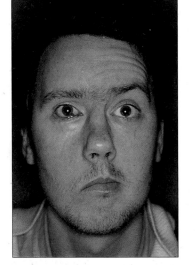

Figure 12.9
Right lower motor neurone facial palsy

narrow the palpebral fissure is usually indicated in high risk or established cases of exposure keratitis.

Other conditions

HORNER'S SYNDROME

Interruption of the sympathetic supply to the eye at any point along its course will lead to ipsilateral ptosis and miosis (small pupil) together referred to as Horner's syndrome (Fig. 12.10). The ptosis is fairly small, no more than 2 mm. The difference in pupil size (anisocoria) is more obvious if the pupils are viewed in dim light when the dilator pupillae muscle causes pupil dilatation.

Causes include the following:

- Within the central nervous system: brainstem CVA, demyelination, tumour
- Proximal to the superior cervical ganglion: apical lung tumour (Pancoast syndrome), cervical rib, tumour
- Distal to the superior cervical ganglion (postganglionic): trauma, carotid artery aneurysm.

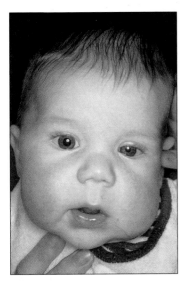

Figure 12.10
Horner's syndrome, left side

ADIE'S SYNDROME

Sudden interruption of the postganglionic parasympathetic supply to the constrictor pupillae muscle causes pupil dilatation and blurred vision due to paralysis of accommodation. The cause of the disease is unknown. Occasionally the pupil lesion may be associated with absence of knee or ankle jerks in Adie's syndrome.

MYASTHENIA GRAVIS

Myasthenia gravis is a chronic neuromuscular disease characterised by excessive fatigability. The extraocular muscles, levator palpebrae superioris and orbicularis oculi may be involved alone (ocular myasthenia), but it is more commonly associated with generalised muscle abnormality. It is an autoimmune condition that targets acetylcholine receptors on striated muscle.

Clinically patients complain of ptosis which worsens during the day, and variable diplopia due to extraocular muscle involvement.

Investigation and treatment

Acetylcholine receptor antibodies are found in 90 per cent of patients. Diagnosis may be confirmed by electromyogram or by the Tensilon test in which there is transient reversal of clinical findings after an intravenous injection of edrophonium bromide (Tensilon). Myasthenia gravis is usually treated with oral anticholinesterases but it may also respond to immunosuppressives or surgical thymectomy.

13 Strabismus (squint)

Anatomy

The following six extraocular muscles in each eye are responsible for eye movements (Figs 13.1 and 13.2).

Superior rectus ⎫
Inferior rectus ⎪ All supplied by the oculomotor nerve
Medial rectus ⎬ (IIIrd cranial nerve)
Inferior oblique ⎭

Superior oblique — Supplied by trochlear nerve (IVth cranial nerve)

Lateral rectus — Supplied by abducent nerve (VIth cranial nerve)

Before describing, defining and classifying the various types of squint it is necessary to describe the normal eye movements.

- **Abduction** the outward movement of the eye
- **Adduction** the inward movement of the eye
- **Conjugate** or **version** movements when the eyes move together in parallel, i.e. looking to the left (laevoversion), looking to the right (dextroversion) or looking up, down or obliquely
- **Disjunctive** or **vergence** movements when the eyes do not move together in parallel but their visual axes come together at a near point such as a book (convergence), or deviate outwards symmetrically (divergence) when asleep or under sedation.

Each ocular muscle is linked with a muscle in the other eye responsible for moving the eyes in a complementary direction ('yoke muscles'). For example the right medial rectus and left lateral rectus are yoke muscles; they are used together in left gaze. Any paralysis of one extraocular muscle will usually produce a compensatory over-action in its yoke muscle.

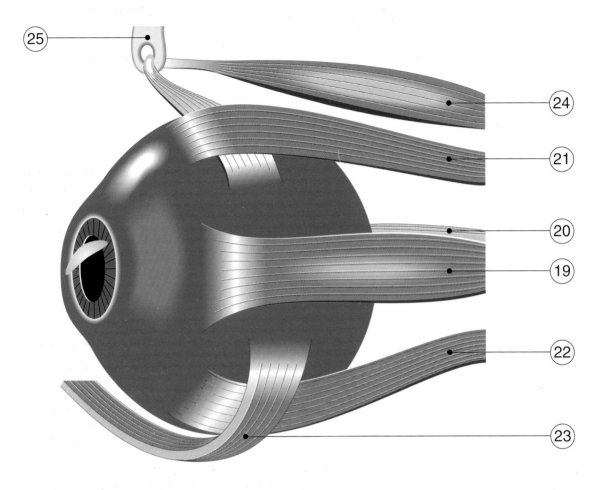

Extrinsic muscles of the eye

19 Lateral rectus
20 Medial rectus
21 Superior rectus
22 Inferior rectus

23 Inferior oblique
24 Superior oblique
25 Trochlea

Figure 13.1
Extraocular (extrinsic) muscles.
(Reproduced with kind
permission of Hoya Corporation,
Japan)

Definition

In strabismus or squint the visual axes of the two eyes are misaligned. The direction of deviation may be horizontal, vertical or torsional or have elements of all these problems. An apparent strabismus (pseudosquint) occurs when there is an appearance of squint but no ocular deviation is demon-

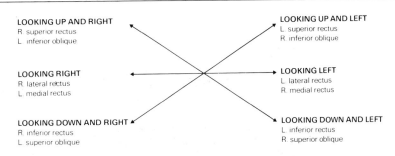

LOOKING UP AND RIGHT
R. superior rectus
L. inferior oblique

LOOKING UP AND LEFT
L. superior rectus
R. inferior oblique

LOOKING RIGHT
R. lateral rectus
L. medial rectus

LOOKING LEFT
L. lateral rectus
R. medial rectus

LOOKING DOWN AND RIGHT
R. inferior rectus
L. superior oblique

LOOKING DOWN AND LEFT
L. inferior rectus
R. superior oblique

Figure 13.2
Principal movement of each
extraocular muscle

strated. In children this is commonly associated with epicanthic folds which are semilunar folds of skin on the medial corner of the eye (Fig. 5.9). These usually reduce in size as the facial structure and the bridge of the nose develop with age.

Classification of squint

A **manifest** squint (tropia) is present all the time, whilst a **latent** squint (phoria) is only present on dissociation of the eyes (see cover test below). Squints vary in direction of deviation:

- Esophoria and esotropia (latent and manifest convergent squint): the deviating eye turns inward (Fig. 13.3)
- Exophoria and exotropia (latent and manifest divergent squint): the deviating eye turns outward (Fig. 13.4)
- Hyperphoria and hypertropia (latent and manifest vertical squint): the deviating eye turns upward
- Hypophoria and hypotropia (latent and manifest vertical squint): the deviating eye turns downward.

In a **concomitant strabismus** (non-paralytic squint) the angle of deviation remains the same in all directions of gaze and the ocular movements are full in all directions. It is the commonest type of squint occurring in children.

In an **incomitant strabismus** the angle of squint varies with the direction of gaze. When secondary to a cranial nerve palsy the squint is maximum when looking in the direction of action of the paralysed muscle.

AETIOLOGY OF CONCOMITANT STRABISMUS

- Genetic factors: 25 per cent of children with squint have a family history of strabismus

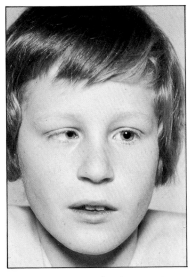

Figure 13.3
Corneal reflections observed in a child with a convergent squint

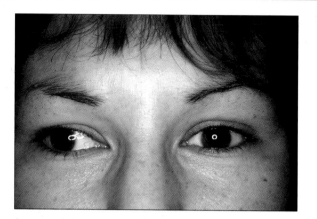

Figure 13.4
Divergent strabismus (Courtesy
of Western Ophthalmic Hospital)

- High refractive errors may be associated with concomitant strabismus and are often inherited
- All children with neurological syndromes and those with multiple handicaps have an increased risk of developing a squint; 50 per cent of children with cerebral palsy have a squint
- Prematurity
- Secondary to poor vision: this may be due to any structural abnormality of the eyes such as persistent hyperplastic primary vitreous, cataract, retinoblastoma, coloboma, or optic nerve abnormality.

AETIOLOGY OF INCOMITANT STRABISMUS

- Congenital abnormalities of muscle or its innervation: **Duane's syndrome** is a horizontal motility defect characterised by variable deficiency of abduction and adduction and palpebral fissure changes, with narrowing on adduction and widening on abduction, and is thought to be due to abnormal innervation of the lateral rectus muscle; **Brown's syndrome** (superior oblique tendon sheath syndrome) is a congenital anomaly of the superior oblique tendon that prevents elevation of the eye in adduction
- Cranial nerve palsies: see Chapter 12
- Muscular disorders: myasthenia gravis, thyroid eye disease (see Chapters 12 and 15 respectively)
- Trauma: particularly following orbital floor ('blow out') fracture where there is limitation of upgaze due to tethering of ocular tissue in the fracture site (see Chapter 8).

Effects of strabismus and amblyopia

In a child strabismus can adversely affect normal visual development because this requires the visual cortex to receive clear, aligned images from each eye. If the visual cortex receives a blurred or misaligned image from one eye it will tend to 'ignore' (suppress) the visual information from that eye and devote an increased proportion of the visual cortex to images received from the 'good' eye. Clinically this is manifest as reduced visual acuity in the affected eye known as **amblyopia** ('lazy eye'). Amblyopia is the commonest visual disability in children and is usually uniocular, although it can occur bilaterally. The commonest cause is squint (**strabismic amblyopia**). Other causes are significant refractive errors and media opacities, where amblyopia develops in the presence of normally aligned eyes ('straight-eyed amblyopia'). The most common cause of straight-eyed amblyopia is **anisometropic amblyopia** which occurs when there is a difference in the refractive error between the two eyes. The eye with the higher refractive error produces a blurred image which is suppressed by the visual cortex.

Amblyopia is potentially reversible particularly if it is identified and treatment commenced at an early age. Once visual maturity has been reached (at 7 or 8 years of age), treatment is ineffective. Early effective treatment may become extremely important for a child in later life especially if the 'good' eye loses vision. Patients with amblyopia have poor vision in one eye and do not develop normal binocular single vision which will prevent them from pursuing certain professions (e.g. HGV driving) in adulthood.

In an adult sudden onset of a squint will not damage the sight but will cause diplopia (double vision). Children who develop a squint before the age of 8 years will tend to suppress the image from the squinting eye, and therefore rarely complain of diplopia.

Management

History

History taking should include a birth history, general health and any medication. A family history of squint or high refractive errors should be sought. Parents should be asked the nature of the squint and when it was first noticed.

Examination

- The examination starts with an **external examination of the face and orbits**, looking for abnormalities or asymmetry.
- **Visual acuity** may be difficult to check accurately in young children, but there are a number of techniques that are available. These include forced choice preferential looking or Cardiff picture cards which do not require any verbal co-operation from the child. As the child grows older, the Kay picture cards and the Sheridan–Gardiner test can be used. In the older child a Snellen chart can be achieved.
- **Cover/uncover and alternate cover tests** are performed to confirm the presence of a squint, check for amblyopia and to differentiate between a latent and a manifest squint respectively. **A cover test** will demonstrate a manifest squint (Figs 13.5 a and b). Each eye is covered in turn as the eyes fix on a target for near and then for distance vision. If the non-fixing (squinting) eye is covered or uncovered there will be no deviation of either eye (Fig. 13.6a). However when the fixing (non-squinting) eye is covered, the squinting eye will have to move to take up fixation. The direction of movement to take up fixation will depend on the type of squint. If the eye is convergent the squinting eye will have to move outwards to take up fixation, and if the deviation is divergent the squinting eye will have to move inwards to take up fixation. As movement of one eye is always associated by an equal and opposite movement of the other eye the eye now under cover will move by a similar amount in the opposite direction (Fig. 13.6b). When the cover is removed (**uncover test**) there are two important possible outcomes. The original fixing eye may resume fixation and the squint will be manifest in the original squinting eye; this suggests that the vision in the squinting eye is worse than in the non-squinting eye, as a patient will generally prefer to fix with the eye with best vision (Fig. 13.6c). Alternatively the eye that was originally squinting remains fixing and the other eye now has a manifest squint; this is known as an alternating squint, and occurs when the vision is equal in both eyes. In an **alternate cover test** the

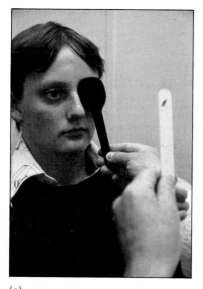

(a)

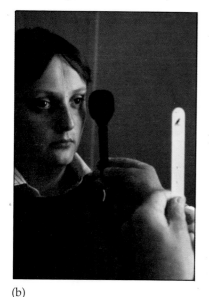

(b)

Figures 13.5 a and b
The cover/uncover test

cover is moved rapidly between the eyes to dissociate them to check for the presence of a latent squint. Again the eyes will move outwards or inwards to take up fixation depending on whether a convergent or divergent phoria or latent squint is present (Fig. 13.7).

- **Ocular movements** should be examined to check for a full range of movements and to differentiate concomitant from incomitant squints.
- Tests for **binocular function** are performed to assess stereopsis or three-dimensional vision.
- **Fundoscopy** and assessment of the ocular media are important to exclude any organic cause for squint such as cataract, retinoblastoma and papilloedema (particularly in patients with a sudden onset of a VIth nerve palsy). Children will usually require to be dilated, most commonly with cyclopentolate 1%. If the eyes are very dark atropine will need to be used for 3 days prior to the appointment to dilate the pupils.
- **Refraction** is an important part of the examination as the provision of spectacles may not only help the treatment of amblyopia but may aid control of the squint. Hypermetropic glasses are helpful in controlling a convergent squint, and myopic glasses can aid control of a divergent squint.

Treatment

This involves excluding and treating any underlying cause, achieving the best possible vision, treating any amblyopia and straightening the eyes.

- Provision of correct glasses, which should be worn full time in children.
- Occlusion therapy, used to reverse amblyopia. The good eye is patched or covered to force the visual input from the poorer eye to be processed by the visual cortex. Patching may vary from a short time such as half an hour each day, to full-time occlusion. Many children are frightened if their good eye is patched particularly if the vision is extremely poor in the amblyopic eye. Although it may be difficult to achieve patching is a vital part of management of a child with amblyopia. In some circumstances the instillation of

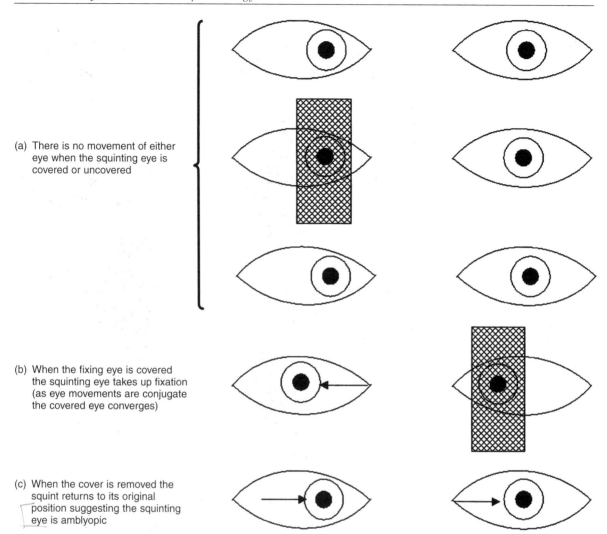

(a) There is no movement of either eye when the squinting eye is covered or uncovered

(b) When the fixing eye is covered the squinting eye takes up fixation (as eye movements are conjugate the covered eye converges)

(c) When the cover is removed the squint returns to its original position suggesting the squinting eye is amblyopic

Figure 13.6
Diagram of cover/uncover test of a manifest convergent squint (esotropia)

atropine drops into the better eye may be useful in those with milder degrees of amblyopia. This works by dilating and blurring vision in the good eye, allowing the weaker eye to do the work.

• Squint surgery should be considered after amblyopia has been treated, when the vision is equal in each eye and the squint alternates freely between each eye. Surgery can be cosmetic, functional or both. The choice of surgical procedure is decided by the type of squint, the angle of squint and the extent of binocular vision. Surgery may be performed on one or both eyes. Muscles can be weakened by recessing them or strengthened by shortening or resecting them. For example with a convergent squint the

(a) There is no movement of either eye during cover/uncover test on either side

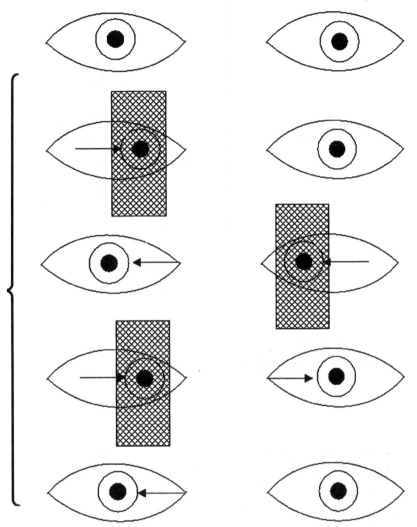

(b) When the cover is alternated between the eyes the eyes are 'dissociated' and the eye under the cover converges and has to move outwards when uncovered to regain fixation

Figure 13.7
Diagram of alternate cover test of a latent convergent squint (esophoria)

medial rectus might be recessed and the lateral rectus resected in one eye, or the medial rectus be recessed in each eye.

- In an adult recent onset of a squint will cause diplopia. This may be overcome with prisms applied to the spectacle lens, by patching the eye or by fogging one spectacle lens. Once the squint is stable then surgery to align the eyes and eliminate diplopia may be considered. In selected patients treatment with **botulinum toxin** may be injected into an overacting muscle to give temporary reversal of a squint and relief of diplopia. This may be particularly useful in treatment of a VIth nerve palsy.

14 Paediatric ophthalmology

Most ophthalmic conditions occur either in paediatric or geriatric patients and although the pathological condition may be the same the impact of the disorder will obviously be different on the young patient with a developing visual system. Children will often need to be handled differently from adults. Many of the conditions affecting children are covered in other chapters. This chapter looks at congenital, common and important paediatric ocular conditions not covered elsewhere in this book.

Anatomy and development

The optic nerve, retina and uvea (consisting of the iris, ciliary body and choroid) develop from a balloon-like outgrowth of the developing brain (optic vesicle). The cornea and lens are derived from surface ectoderm. The developing lens indents the optic vesicle which invaginates into a cup shape that eventually fuses inferiorly along the choroidal fissure. An artery passes through the early vitreous to supply the lens but this atrophies and the lens becomes avascular. The surface ectoderm separates into the cornea and lens and the cleft between the two develops to form the anterior chamber.

In dealing with paediatric ophthalmological problems it is important to remember that the visual system in a child goes through various periods of development until it reaches maturity. In the first 6 weeks of life there is a latent period when visual deprivation does not appear to significantly affect long-term visual outcome. Thereafter there follows a critical or sensitive period lasting until the age of 8 years during which time any disease process can have a damaging effect on the development of sight (amblyopia; see Chapter 13).

Paediatric conditions will be discussed under the following headings:

- Congenital anomalies
- Watery and sticky eyes
- Orbital cellulitis
- Leukocoria.

Congenital anomalies

PTOSIS

Causes

- An isolated congenital defect is due to incomplete development (dystrophy) of the levator palpebrae superioris muscle, which may rarely be associated with a defect of the superior rectus muscle preventing elevation of the eye (Fig. 14.1)
- In congenital IIIrd nerve palsy there is the characteristic ocular motility defect and there may be pupil involvement
- In congenital Horner's syndrome the ptosis is slight and is associated with heterochromia of the iris and a small pupil
- In Marcus–Gunn (jaw-winking) syndrome the ptosis varies with sucking or chewing due to an innervation abnormality.

Treatment

A complete ptosis requires urgent management to prevent severe amblyopia. Children with partial ptosis require careful monitoring for amblyopia and astigmatic refractive errors caused by lid pressure on the developing globe. Early surgery is necessary if the vision is affected; otherwise corrective repair is left until the child is over 4 years old.

CAPILLARY HAEMANGIOMA OR STRAWBERRY NAEVUS

This is a benign neoplasm of abnormal blood vessels (Fig. 14.2) and is usually noticed at birth, increases in size and then spontaneously regresses. It is most commonly found in the upper lid or orbit. A capillary haemangioma of the orbit will present as proptosis. If the upper lid is affected and there is

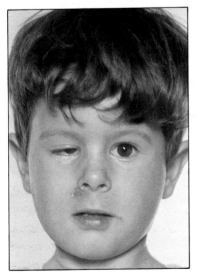

Figure 14.1
Congenital ptosis

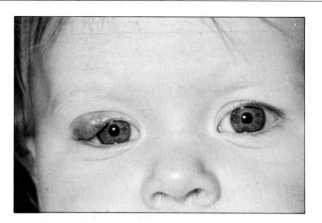

Figure 14.2
Haemangioma of the eyelid

significant ptosis vision can be markedly reduced due to amblyopia. As the tumour will regress active treatment is only necessary if the visual axis is occluded. Treatment is usually given in the form of a local injection of steroid. Surgical debulking is not advised.

DERMOIDS

These are congenital overgrowths of surface ectoderm that become sequestered in embryonic lines of closure. They present as subcutaneous firm, smooth, swellings usually at the lateral aspect of the upper lid. Care must be taken when excision is planned as they may extend posteriorly into the deeper orbital structures. Rupture may produce a severe inflammatory reaction. Rarely a dermoid may be found at the corneoscleral junction of the eye.

COLOBOMA

A coloboma results from failure of closure of the choroidal fissure of the embryonic optic cup. Anterior lesions affect the ciliary body, iris and/or lens, whereas posterior lesions affect the choroid and retina. As the choroidal fissure closes inferiorly colobomata generally occur inferiorly.

An anterior coloboma usually presents as a cat's eye or keyhole shaped pupil (Fig. 14.3). A small posterior coloboma is often asymptomatic and may be an incidental finding or noticed as a field defect on routine testing in later life. A large or posterior chorioretinal coloboma may present in childhood as a squint, poor vision, or rarely as leukocoria.

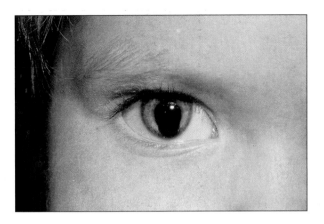

Figure 14.3
Coloboma of iris

CONGENITAL CATARACT

See Chapter 9.

Sticky and watery eyes

NEONATAL CONJUNCTIVITIS (OPHTHALMIA NEONATORUM)

Ocular infection occurring during passage of the infant through an infected birth canal may cause a severe purulent conjunctivitis known as ophthalmia neonatorum, usually occurring 2–10 days after birth. The most commonly identified causative organism is *Chlamydia trachomatis*, with other causes of infection being staphylococcus and *E. coli*. Ophthalmia neonatorum caused by *Neisseria gonorrhoeae* is a rare but potentially devastating infection, causing a severe purulent conjunctivitis with the risk of corneal infection and perforation. It is important to consider all purulent conjunctivitis occurring in the first few days of life as gonococcal until proved otherwise. Investigations should include conjunctival swabs and Gram stain of conjunctival scrapings. Children at high risk or with proven gonoccocal conjunctivitis should be hospitalised and treated with high-dose parenteral and topical penicillin. Chlamydia infection requires systemic treatment with erythromycin. In gonococcal or chlamydial infection the parents need investigation and treatment for genital infection.

CONGENITAL NASOLACRIMAL DUCT OBSTRUCTION

Unilateral or bilateral sticky eyes in babies during the first few months of life are frequently caused by late opening or canalisation of the lower end of the nasolacrimal duct. Delayed opening of the duct may be recognised by watering eyes in the baby from soon after birth, or from intermittent or persistent episodes of recurrent infection. The eyes usually remain white. Pressure over the nasolacrimal region produces regurgitation of pus and mucus. Most cases will resolve spontaneously with complete opening of the lower end of the nasolacrimal duct. Treatment is therefore expectant, with cleaning of the eye with sterile water and massage over the nasolacrimal sac to express stagnant secretions and encourage canalisation. Poor tear drainage leads to an increased incidence of infections which may need treating with antibiotic eye drops. Probing of the nasolacrimal system under general anaesthetic is only considered if the situation has not resolved once the child is 1 year old.

CONJUNCTIVITIS ASSOCIATED WITH UPPER RESPIRATORY TRACT INFECTION

When a child gets an upper respiratory tract infection there is nasal blockage with conjunctivitis. It is treated with topical antibiotics and nasal decongestants and does not require syringing and probing.

CONGENITAL GLAUCOMA

Epiphora is a common symptom in congenital glaucoma (see Chapter 10).

Orbital cellulitis

This is a serious sight- and life-threatening condition. Inflammation of the orbital tissues is usually caused by spread of infection from adjacent structures, most commonly from the paranasal air sinuses (especially the thin ethmoidal sinuses). Injury to the orbit may also introduce infection. It is most commonly seen in children and young adults. Sight may be threatened due to raised orbital pressure which may damage the optic nerve. Spread of infection posteriorly into the brain may be potentially life-threatening.

Signs and symptoms

- Unwell and febrile patient
- Periorbital redness, swelling and pain (Fig. 14.4)
- Proptosis
- Reduced visual acuity
- Red, chemosed conjunctiva
- Impaired ocular movements
- Relative afferent pupil defect
- Reduced colour vision (especially red, suggesting optic nerve compression)
- Swollen optic disc.

It is important to realise that most patients will not have all of these signs and symptoms particularly in the early stages. A cellulitis around the eye should be treated as orbital cellulitis if there is any suggestion of ocular dysfunction as described above.

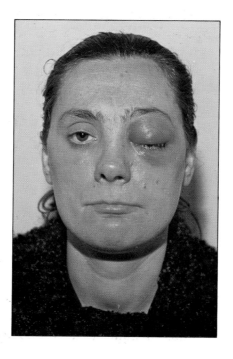

Figure 14.4
Orbital cellulitis

Treatment

The patient should be admitted for blood cultures and intravenous antibiotics. Sinus X-rays and an ENT opinion are usually required. Surgical drainage of the sinuses or a localised orbital abscess may be necessary.

PRE-SEPTAL CELLULITIS

Pre-septal cellulitis is present if infection is in the skin and soft tissues and has not spread through the orbital septum into the orbit. It is essentially a skin cellulitis and the eye is therefore not affected. Pre-septal cellulitis may follow an infected chalazion, skin lesion or an upper respiratory tract infection. The patient has a swollen lid but the vision is normal, the eye is not proptosed and there is no limitation of ocular movement. Treatment is with systemic antibiotics.

Leukocoria

Leukocoria or white pupil is an important and serious sign in a child (Fig. 14.5). It requires urgent referral for specialist evaluation and differential diagnosis.

RETINOBLASTOMA

Retinoblastoma is the commonest malignant ocular tumour of childhood, occurring in 1 in 20 000 live births. The child will die without treatment but a high survival rate is achiev-

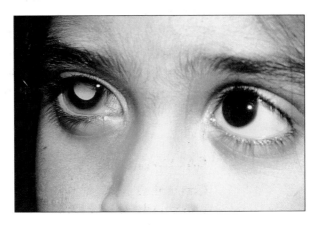

Figure 14.5
Leukocoria

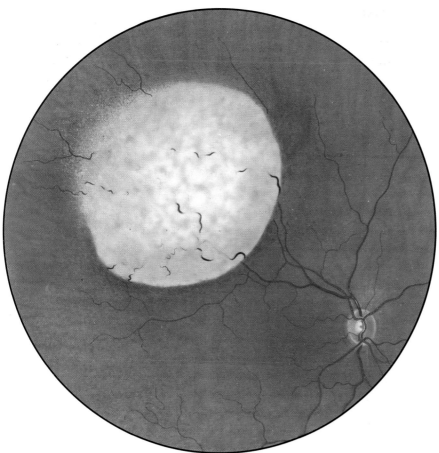

Figure 14.6
Retinoblastoma

able with treatment. It is a malignant tumour of embryonic retinal cells and in 90 per cent of cases, presents in a child less than 3 years of age. Most children with retinoblastoma present with leukocoria and/or squint. The ophthalmoscopic appearance is of a raised, white area in the fundus of the infant (Fig. 14.6). The tumour may be single, multiple or bilateral. Multiple or bilateral tumours indicate a hereditary cause. Methods of treatment include enucleation, irradiation, chemotherapy and cryotherapy. With modern methods of treatment the prognosis is excellent.

CATARACT

Congenital cataract may present with a white pupil either uniocularly or bilaterally.

RETINOPATHY OF PREMATURITY (ROP)

ROP is a multifactorial disease that occurs in the smallest and sickest premature babies. Babies of less than 31 weeks, gestation and weighing less than 1501 g are screened for ROP. The majority of ROP is mild and regresses spontaneously with time having no long-term effect on vision. Severe ROP can often be successfully treated using retinal cryotherapy or laser. Despite treatment there is still a failure rate with some children going blind due to retinal detachment. The fibrosed retina forms a retrolental membrane giving the appearance of a white pupil. Although severe ROP in older neonates has markedly reduced due to improvements in neonatal care the overall incidence is increasing due to the increased survival rate of extremely premature babies.

PERSISTENT HYPERPLASTIC PRIMARY VITREOUS (PHPV)

PHPV is a congenital abnormality of the eye in which the vitreous does not develop normally. It is usually unilateral and presents with a white pupil and a small eye. There is a stalk of fibrous tissue from the posterior pole of the retina to the back of the lens and the diagnosis can be confirmed with an ultrasound scan.

COLOBOMA

A large posterior coloboma may present as leukocoria.

15

Ocular manifestations of systemic disease

The recognition of certain ocular signs and symptoms may often be of value in establishing a diagnosis or assessing the severity of a systemic disorder. A wide range of systemic conditions will be discussed in this chapter; many are common but some are rare with important or characteristic ocular features. The systemic conditions in this chapter will be described under the following group headings:

- Endocrine disease
- Vascular and haematological disease
- Rheumatic disease
- Infectious and granulomatous disease
- Skin and mucous membrane disease
- Genetic disease.

Endocrine disease

DIABETES

Diabetic patients are prone to a fluctuating refractive error (due to osmotic changes in lens hydration with varying blood sugar), eyelid styes, the formation of eyelid xanthelasma, earlier development of cataracts, chronic open angle glaucoma, cranial nerve palsies, ischaemic optic neuropathy and retinal vascular occlusions. The most serious ocular complication is **diabetic retinopathy** which is the commonest cause of blindness in adults under 65 years of age in the developed world.

The development of diabetic retinopathy is related to two factors:

- The **duration** of diabetes; diabetic retinopathy may be observed in approximately 80 per cent of diabetics after 20 years of the disease.

- The **control** of the diabetes; adequate control delays the onset and slows the progression of diabetic retinopathy.

Diabetic retinopathy is a microvascular disease, caused by occlusion of retinal capillaries and leakage of plasma contents into the retina.

CLASSIFICATION OF DIABETIC RETINOPATHY

- **Non-proliferative (background) diabetic retinopathy**. This covers a wide range of diabetic retinopathy from mild background retinopathy to severe pre-proliferative disease. Microaneurysms are the earliest visible changes, followed by retinal oedema, hard exudate and flame-shaped haemorrhages (Fig. 15.1). The development of cotton wool spots, deep blot haemorrhages and retinal venous changes indicates the presence of retinal ischaemia.
- **Proliferative diabetic retinopathy**. Marked retinal ischaemia leads to the development of new retinal vessels (neovascularisation). This is most commonly seen on the optic nerve head (Fig. 15.2) but may also occur elsewhere on the retina or on the iris. The new vessels are fragile and may bleed into the vitreous causing loss of sight. Scar tissue associated with the new vessels can lead to tractional retinal detachment. Proliferative retinopathy is commoner in insulin dependent (type 1) diabetics. If untreated 50 per cent of eyes with new vessels will become blind in 5 years.
- **Diabetic maculopathy**. This term describes macular

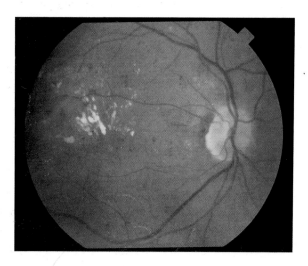

Figure 15.1
Moderate background diabetic retinopathy affecting macular region (diabetic maculopathy)

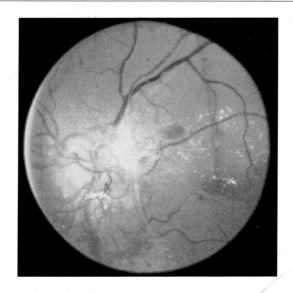

Figure 15.2
Proliferative diabetic retinopathy
with fibrovascular tissue around
optic disc

involvement with microaneurysms, haemorrhage, oedema, exudate or ischaemia. It can occur in combination with other types of retinopathy and is associated with a high incidence of visual loss being the commonest cause of diabetic blindness. It is commoner in type II (non-insulin dependent) diabetics.

Symptoms

Diabetic retinopathy is asymptomatic unless the macula is involved or new vessels bleed causing vitreous haemorrhage with sudden loss of sight. Because of this diabetics should have regular fundus examinations, especially in pregnancy when diabetic retinopathy may progress rapidly.

Treatment

Good diabetic control may delay the development and lessen the severity of diabetic retinopathy. Hypertension and hyperlipidaemia may worsen diabetic retinopathy and should be controlled.

Treatment may be by the following methods:

- **Laser**. Diabetic maculopathy may be treated by the application of a small number of laser burns around the macula to seal the leaking blood vessels (focal laser). Proliferative diabetic retinopathy is treated by extensively lasering the ischaemic peripheral retina (panretinal photocoagulation) which reduces the drive to new blood vessel formation and causes regression of new vessels. Laser treatment is usually performed as an out-patient procedure and repeated photocoagulation is frequently required.

- **Surgery**. Diabetic patients with non-clearing vitreous haemorrhage or tractional retinal detachment threatening the macula may be treated by vitrectomy where the vitreous and any associated haemorrhage or fibrous tissue is removed.

THYROID DISEASE

Disorders of the thyroid gland are frequently associated with ocular signs and symptoms. Untreated hyperthyroidism (thyrotoxicosis) often causes upper lid retraction, giving the appearance of 'staring eyes'. These signs arise from excessive stimulation of the smooth muscle part of the levator palpebrae superioris (Müller's muscle) and settle rapidly on returning to the euthyroid state. Untreated hypothyroidism (myxoedema) is associated with periorbital oedema (Fig. 15.3) and loss of eyebrow hair (madarosis).

THYROID EYE DISEASE (DYSTHYROID EYE DISEASE; OPHTHALMIC GRAVES' DISEASE)

Autoimmune hyperthyroidism (Graves' disease) is the commonest form of hyperthyroidism. The autoimmune process may cause inflammation and swelling of orbital structures (particularly extraocular muscles), leading to

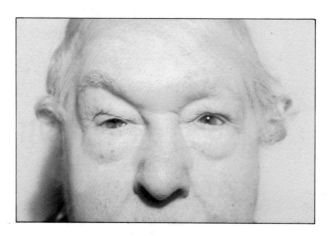

Figure 15.3
Hypothyroidism

proptosis (or exophthalmos) and rarely optic nerve compression. In severe cases the eyes can become so proptosed that the lids cannot adequately cover the cornea and exposure keratitis may develop. Extraocular muscle involvement frequently causes incomitant strabismus and diplopia (Fig. 15.4).

Although usually bilateral thyroid eye disease may be markedly asymmetric and indeed is the commonest cause of a unilateral proptosis.

Treatment

If patients are thyrotoxic this should be normalised, but hypothyroidism must be avoided as this may exacerbate the eye problems. Thyroid eye disease usually has an active phase of orbital inflammation that may last for several years followed by a quiescent ('burnt out') phase where fibrotic changes within muscles become more significant. It is felt that the degree of fibrotic change is related to the severity of the inflammatory phase and that reducing the severity of inflammation during the active phase may lead to less severe fibrotic changes. Treatment of the active phase ranges from simple lubricating eye drops to systemic immunosuppressives, orbital radiotherapy and surgical procedures such as tarsorrhaphy and orbital decompression, depending on the severity of disease. Diplopia is treated with prisms during the active phase as surgery is very unpredictable in the face of active inflammation. In the quiescent phase muscle surgery may be used to alleviate diplopia and upper lid lowering and

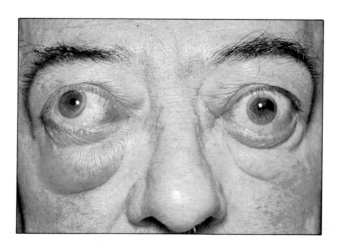

Figure 15.4
Thyrotoxicosis with exophthalmos, eyelid retraction and defective eye movement

orbital decompression may be used to improve the cosmetic appearance of the eyes.

PARATHYROID DISEASE

Hyperparathyroidism leads to hypercalcaemia which may cause calcium salts to deposit in the corneal stroma in a band-like fashion (band keratopathy). Hypoparathyroidism leads to hypocalcaemia, which may be associated with congenital or early onset cataract.

PITUITARY TUMOURS

Pituitary adenomas are the commonest cause of pituitary disease and cause endocrine problems either by excessive or inadequate hormone production from the remaining normal pituitary gland. Pituitary adenomas tend to expand superiorly and encroach on the optic chiasma causing a bitemporal hemianopia (see Chapter 12).

Vascular and haematological disease

HYPERTENSION

High blood pressure is associated with cranial nerve palsies and retinal vascular disease.

HYPERTENSIVE RETINOPATHY

Systemic hypertension whatever the cause may produce important diagnostic fundus appearances. The ocular appearances depend on the severity and duration of the blood pressure elevation. Only an acute severe rise (grades III or IV, see below) in blood pressure causes visual symptoms; less severe degrees are asymptomatic.

Clinical features

In the face of increased blood pressure retinal arterioles vasoconstrict and this appears clinically as arteriolar

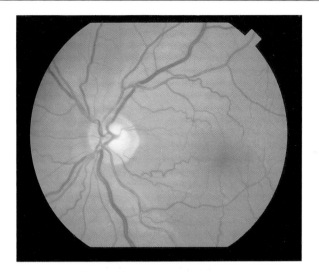

Figure 15.5
Early hypertension: note
arteriovenous (AV) nipping and
arteriolar narrowing

attenuation (Fig. 15.5). Prolonged hypertension causes vessel wall thickening which appears ophthalmoscopically as a reduced redness and increased light reflex of arterioles, so-called copper or (if more advanced) silver wiring. Arteriovenous nipping of the venules occurs where thickened arterioles compress an underlying vein thus tapering off the column of blood in that part of the vein. Capillary leakage may occur if blood pressure is acutely markedly raised and causes retinal flame haemorrhages, oedema, hard exudates and optic nerve swelling (Figs 15.6 and 15.7). Cotton wool spots are evidence of retinal ischaemia representing the interruption of axoplasmic flow in the retinal nerve fibres.

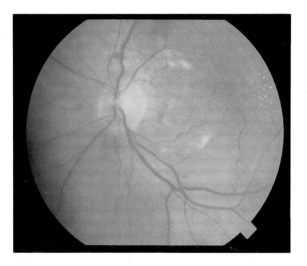

Figure 15.6
Moderate hypertension: note
haemorrhages and cotton wool
spots

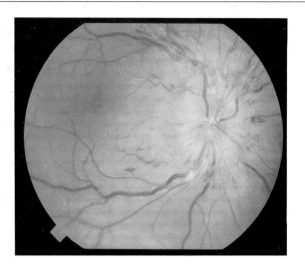

Figure 15.7
Severe hypertension: note the swollen disc in addition to vessel changes and haemorrhages

Grading

Grade I (mild hypertension)	Arteriolar attenuation, copper wiring
Grade II (moderate hypertension)	AV nipping, silver wiring, occasional hard exudate or haemorrhage
Grade III (severe hypertension)	Flame haemorrhages, hard exudates, cotton wool spots
Grade IV (malignant hypertension)	as for grade III, with disc swelling

Treatment

Grades III and IV can usually be reversed by adequate blood pressure control. Grades I and II are more resistant to reversal, even if blood pressure is normalised.

ATHEROMA

Atheroma may cause ophthalmic disease by embolisation, or by directly interfering with ocular or cerebral perfusion.

- **Embolisation**. Emboli affecting the ocular circulation most commonly arise from atheromatous plaques at the origin of the internal carotid artery or less frequently from a mural thrombus or calcified aortic valve. Such emboli may temporarily occlude the central retinal artery causing a transient loss of vision (**amaurosis fugax**), or they may permanently occlude the central retinal artery or one of its branches (central or branch retinal artery occlusion; see Chapter 11). Amaurosis fugax typically causes monocular blindness or partial blindness lasting less than 10 minutes and is an important symptom because it is the ocular equivalent of the transient ischaemic attack (TIA) and is associated with an increased risk of stroke. Temporal arteritis may mimic the symptoms of amaurosis fugax and it is essential that all such patients should have this diagnosis excluded. Patients suffering an attack of amaurosis fugax or retinal artery occlusion should be assessed to identify possible risk factors and sources of emboli.

- **Vertebrobasilar insufficiency**. Ischaemia of the occipital cortex may produce transient visual symptoms including blindness and hemianopia or other field loss. This may be produced by a stenosed vertebrobasilar artery or by mechanical obstruction of vertebral arteries as they ascend a degenerative vertebral column in certain neck positions.

ANAEMIA

The commonest ocular finding in anaemia is pallor of the inferior tarsal conjunctiva. Flame-shaped retinal nerve fibre layer haemorrhages are the hallmark of anaemic retinopathy and they are only found in the presence of severe anaemia. Cotton wool spots are a less frequent observation.

- **Pernicious anaemia**. This is caused by vitamin B12 deficiency and may be associated with an optic neuropathy. There is typically loss of central vision and a reduction in colour vision in association with optic atrophy. The condition may be arrested by periodic intramuscular injections of hydroxocobalamin.
- **Sickle cell anaemia**. This is a group of disorders in which normal adult haemoglobin (HbA) is replaced with a variant such as HbS or HbC causing increased blood viscosity, anaemia and vascular occlusion. Although sickle cell haemoglobin S disease has more systemic manifestations, sickle cell haemoglobin C disease has more severe ocular complications. Ocular findings include large intraretinal haemorrhage (salmon patch) and 'black sunbursts' which

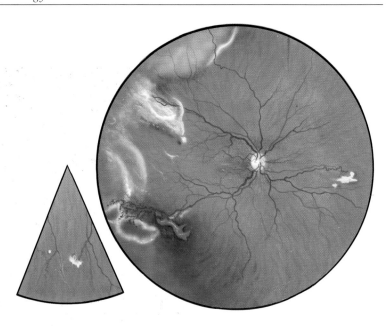

Figure 15.8
Fundus in sickle cell disease

are chorioretinal scars following the retinal haemorrhages. The most serious complication is proliferative retinopathy with neovascular tissue described as 'sea fans' developing at the junction of ischaemic and non-ischaemic retina (Fig. 15.8). These vessels may bleed causing vitreous haemorrhage, traction and retinal detachment. The value of extensive laser is unproven although focal treatment may be helpful. Vitreous haemorrhage or retinal detachment may require surgery.

POLYCYTHAEMIA

Polycythaemia is an abnormal elevation of the red blood cell count. It is an occasional cause of central retinal vein occlusion (see Chapter 11).

LEUKAEMIA

Leukaemia produces a retinopathy identical to that of any severe anaemia, but may also be associated with other ocular features such as uveitis and optic nerve infiltration or proptosis due to orbital infiltration (especially in children) (Fig. 15.9).

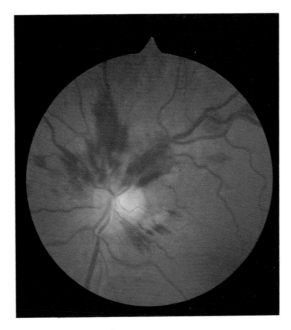

Figure 15.9
Fundus in leukaemia

Rheumatic disease

RHEUMATOID ARTHRITIS

Rheumatoid arthritis is an autoimmune inflammatory joint disease affecting predominantly middle-aged women. A similar inflammatory process may affect the lacrimal gland causing keratoconjunctivitis sicca, or the outer collagenous coats of the eye causing scleritis, episcleritis or keratitis. Keratoconjunctivitis sicca is the most frequent ocular association and occurs in some 10–25 per cent of patients with rheumatoid arthritis.

SJÖGREN'S SYNDROME

Sjögren's syndrome is the name given to the common association of dry eyes (keratoconjunctivitis sicca) and dry mouth (xerostomia). It may occur as an isolated finding (primary Sjögren's) but in the majority of patients it occurs secondary to rheumatoid arthritis.

SYSTEMIC LUPUS ERYTHEMATOSUS (SLE)

This uncommon multisystem disease predominantly affects young black women. It is characterised by the presence in the serum of antinuclear antibodies. The clinical picture of the disease varies enormously but most of the features are due to the consequences of vasculitis.

The common ocular manifestations are keratoconjunctivitis sicca and retinal cotton wool spots which occur secondary to retinal ischaemia.

GIANT CELL/TEMPORAL ARTERITIS AND POLYMYALGIA RHEUMATICA

Temporal (or cranial) arteritis and polymyalgia rheumatica can be regarded as belonging to the same disease spectrum. Polymyalgia rheumatica causes bilateral painful restriction of movement of the shoulders and hips. Temporal arteritis mainly affects women over 70 years who present with malaise and weight loss, jaw claudication, temporal headache and tenderness with thickened temporal arteries (Fig. 15.10). The ESR (erythrocyte sedimentation rate) and C-reactive protein are usually markedly raised.

Ocular complications

- Transient monocular visual loss (amaurosis fugax)
- Visual loss due to central retinal artery occlusion or anterior ischaemic optic neuropathy
- Visual field defects
- Diplopia due to cranial nerve palsy.

Management

Corticosteroid treatment must be started immediately the

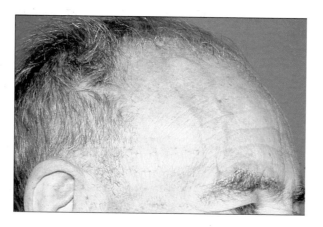

Figure 15.10.
Thickened temporal artery in giant cell arteritis.

diagnosis is suspected (prednisolone 60–80 mg daily). Prompt treatment may prevent visual loss in an eye experiencing amaurosis symptoms. In an eye with sudden visual loss corticosteroid treatment is unlikely to have any effect; however urgent commencement of steroids is essential to reduce the likelihood of second eye involvement which frequently follows the first eye, often in a matter of hours. Temporal artery biopsy may be helpful to confirm the clinical diagnosis. Treatment with steroids will need to be continued for many months.

JUVENILE CHRONIC ARTHRITIS (JUVENILE RHEUMATOID ARTHRITIS)

Chronic arthritis in a patient less than 16 years old is termed juvenile chronic arthritis. It occurs in three forms:

- Arthritis with acute febrile onset, lymphadenopathy and hepatosplenomegaly (Still's disease)
- Polyarticular onset with more than four joints affected
- Pauciarticular onset with less than four joints affected.

Pauciarticular disease in particular is associated with ocular involvement and 20 per cent of patients develop chronic bilateral uveitis. This is frequently complicated by cataract, glaucoma and band keratopathy (calcium deposition in the anterior cornea). Screening of at risk patients is essential as the uveitis is usually asymptomatic.

ANKYLOSING SPONDYLITIS

This disease predominantly affects young men who are positive for the HLA B27 histocompatibility antigen. It causes sacroileitis with lower back pain. Anterior uveitis occurs in approximately 40 per cent of patients and is a recurrent problem. The inflammation is often severe and hypopyon may develop. Ankylosing spondylitis is the commonest systemic association of anterior uveitis.

REITER'S DISEASE

This syndrome typically affects young men who present with conjunctivitis, urethritis, mouth ulcers and arthritis. In children it is associated with a gastrointestinal infection rather than urethritis.

INFLAMMATORY BOWEL DISEASE

Two major forms of inflammatory bowel disease are recognised; Crohn's disease which can affect any part of the gastrointestinal tract, and ulcerative colitis which only affects the large bowel. The most important ophthalmic association is recurrent anterior uveitis which develops in around 5 per cent of patients.

Infectious and granulomatous disease

ACQUIRED IMMUNODEFICIENCY SYNDROME (AIDS)

The acquired immunodeficiency syndrome is caused by the human immunodeficiency virus (HIV) an RNA retrovirus which infects T-helper (CD4+) lymphocytes impairing their function and causing a state of immunodeficiency.

Ocular manifestations

- **Microvascular changes** (**HIV retinopathy**). Cotton wool spots are the most common ocular manifestation of HIV infection. Other less frequently observed changes include retinal haemorrhages, microaneurysms and oedema a picture which may mimic early diabetic retinopathy.
- **Opportunistic ocular infections**. Cytomegalovirus (CMV) retinitis is the most common ocular opportunistic infection seen in AIDS patients. CMV is a member of the herpes group of DNA viruses and causes retinitis in about 25 per cent of AIDS patients. The clinical appearance is of a slowly progressive, necrotising retinitis. White areas of retinal infiltrate and necrosis are associated with retinal haemorrhage within the necrotic area and along the leading edge ('pizza fundus') (Fig. 15.11). Untreated the retinitis slowly progresses, in a 'brush fire' manner, leaving behind atrophic, avascular retina. CMV retinitis is generally asymptomatic until the macula or optic nerve is affected and therefore it is important to screen high-risk patients for asymptomatic disease. Antiviral treatment with ganciclovir

or foscarnet can be given intravenously, by intravitreal injection or implant.

- **Kaposi's sarcoma**. This slowly progressive vascular malignancy is common in AIDS patients. Ocular Kaposi's sarcoma may occur on the eyelids or conjunctiva and appears as a purple/red highly vascular lesion. These lesions are often responsive to radiotherapy.

SEPTICAEMIA

Bacterial septicaemia may occasionally involve the eye and orbit with the development of endophthalmitis or orbital cellulitis respectively. Fungal infections, in particular Candida are an uncommon cause of endophthalmitis, occurring typically in the immunosuppressed or in intravenous drug abusers. Patients with subacute bacterial endocarditis may develop infected microemboli in the retinal circulation which appear clinically as a flame-shaped haemorrhage with a white centre (Roth spot).

SYPHILIS

Syphilis is caused by *Treponema pallidum* and is becoming more common due to the AIDS epidemic.

- **Congenital syphilis**. This characteristically causes a widespread inflammation of the deep corneal stroma known as interstitial keratitis, pigmentary retinopathy ('salt and pepper fundus') and optic atrophy.

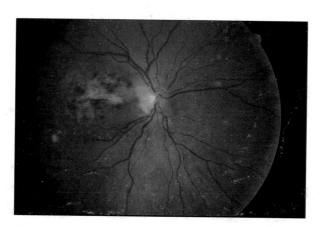

Figure 15.11
Cytomegalovirus retinitis in AIDS ('pizza fundus')

- **Acquired syphilis**. Primary syphilis does not affect the eye. Uveitis and retinitis may occur in the secondary stage of the disease. Tertiary syphilis is now rare but neurosyphilis is associated with ocular features of optic atrophy, cranial nerve palsies and Argyll Robertson pupils (small, irregular pupils that react to accommodation but not to light).

Although rare, syphilis should always be considered in the diagnosis of patients with uveitis or retinitis of unknown cause, as the condition is responsive to treatment with penicillin.

CHLAMYDIAE

Chlamydiae are obligate intracellular bacteria. There are three species although *Chlamydia trachomatis* is the most important with regard to the eye:

- **Ophthalmia neonatorum** (see Chapter 14).
- **Adult inclusion conjunctivitis**. Usually presents as an acute follicular conjunctivitis with mucopurulent discharge and pre-auricular lymphadenopathy in young adults harbouring a genital chlamydia infection.
- **Trachoma**. The commonest cause of preventable blindness world-wide. The disease is spread from eye to eye by common flies. It causes chronic conjunctivitis which eventually leads to entropion, trichiasis, corneal scarring and blindness (Figs 15.12 and 15.13).

Active trachoma may be treated with topical or systemic tetracyclines. Surgery may be useful in correcting entropion

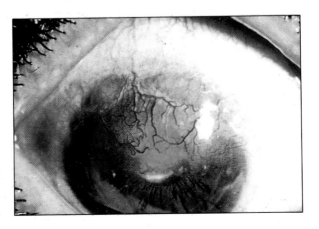

Figure 15.12
Pannus in trachomatous keratitis

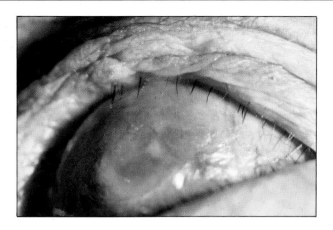

Figure 15.13
Trichiasis and corneal scarring
following trachomatous keratitis

thereby preventing corneal scarring. Corneal grafting may be of use in end-stage disease with corneal scarring.

ONCHOCERCIASIS

Onchocerciasis or river blindness accounts for over 300 000 causes of blindness worldwide. It follows a bite from a fly infected with the nematode *Onchocerca volvulus* which causes the disease. The ocular complications are keratitis, uveitis and optic atrophy.

LEPROSY

Leprosy affects over 15 million people worldwide and has the highest incidence of ocular complications of any systemic disease. Cranial nerve involvement is common in tuberculoid leprosy. Involvement of the Vth cranial nerve may give rise to corneal anaesthesia and neuropathic keratitis, whilst VIIth cranial nerve involvement may lead to ocular complications of facial nerve palsy (ectropion, lagophthalmos, corneal exposure keratopathy). Lepromatous leprosy is typically associated with interstitial keratitis, uveitis and scleritis.

TUBERCULOSIS

Tuberculosis has recently increased in prevalence due to the AIDS epidemic and increasing use of immunosuppressive drugs. The patients may develop a raised pink inflammatory nodule on the conjunctiva with surrounding conjunctival inflammation, so-called phlytenular conjunctivitis. More commonly patients may develop uveitis. Rarely miliary disease may cause multiple small yellow tubercles to develop in the choroid.

SARCOIDOSIS

Sarcoidosis is a multisystem granulomatous disorder of unknown aetiology, but with some similarities to tuberculosis. An infective aetiology has been suspected but never proven. It typically affects young women and is more common in black Americans.

Uveitis develops in around 30 per cent of patients with sarcoidosis and this accounts for 2 per cent of patients with uveitis. Retinal involvement occurs in around 25 per cent of patients with ocular sarcoid. Granulomatous inflammation may affect the lacrimal gland leading to enlargement and keratoconjunctivitis sicca.

Skin and mucous membrane disease

ACNE ROSACEA

This is a chronic inflammatory facial eruption characterised by erythema and telangiectasia. It usually occurs in middle-aged women who often give a history of a ready flushing tendency. Approximately one-half of patients have ocular lesions. Blepharitis and conjunctivitis are common but episcleritis, iritis and keratitis may also occur. Long-term treatment with low-dose systemic tetracycline often improves the inflammatory aspect of the skin and reduces the severity of ocular complications.

PSORIASIS

Although ocular complications are rare with this chronic skin condition 10 per cent of sufferers have an associated arthropathy and these patients may develop acute anterior uveitis.

ATOPIC DERMATITIS (ECZEMA)

Atopic dermatitis most commonly affects the skin creases but in more severely affected patients the face and eyelids can be involved, becoming thickened and excoriated. Atopic dermatitis may also be associated with pre-senile cataract, chronic keratoconjunctivitis and keratoconus.

ALLERGIC DERMATITIS

Due to the laxity of eyelid tissues dramatic and alarming swelling may occur when an allergen precipitates an acute allergic reaction. This may occur as part of a generalised allergic reaction or due to a local contact dermatitis, for example caused by eye drops or make-up. Reassurance and removal of any suspected allergen is usually all that is required. Antihistamines may be of use in the context of a mild generalised allergic reaction, whereas a severe anaphylactic allergic reaction requires emergency resuscitative procedures.

BEHÇET'S SYNDROME

This is a rare condition affecting young adults characterised by oral and genital ulceration, ocular inflammation, arthritis and erythema nodosum. The basis of these manifestations is an obliterative vasculitis. The ocular signs are recurrent hypopyon uveitis, retinal vasculitis and haemorrhage. This is a potentially blinding disease that requires systemic immunosuppressive treatment.

OCULAR PEMPHIGOID

'Benign mucous membrane pemphigoid' is a rather misleading title for this potentially blinding ocular disorder that affects mainly elderly women. It is characterised by recurrent bullous lesions of the skin and mucous membranes, especially of the mouth and conjunctiva. Ocular involvement presents as a bilateral, chronic conjunctivitis followed by subconjunctival fibrosis with severe tear deficiency, entropion and trichiasis, corneal exposure, opacification and vascularisation (Fig. 15.14). Treatment varies according to the severity and activity of the disease but may involve systemic immunosuppressives.

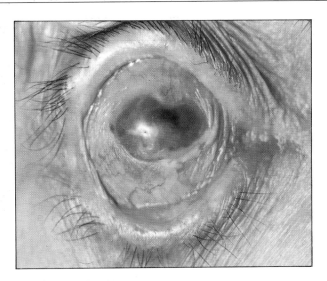

Figure 15.14
Ocular pemphigoid

STEVENS–JOHNSON SYNDROME (ERYTHEMA MULTIFORME)

This is an acute systemic condition characterised by a skin rash and mucous membrane ulceration. It may be caused by a hypersensitive reaction to a drug or follow an infection. Ocular involvement presents as bilateral severe conjunctivitis with subconjunctival scarring. This causes adhesions between the lid and the globe, lid deformities, dry eye and ultimately corneal damage and visual loss. Treatment is with systemic and topical steroids and the relief of forming adhesions.

Genetic disease

The number of inherited systemic disorders with ocular involvement is far too numerous to consider within this text. Below follows a brief outline of disorders with important or characteristic ocular features. Inherited disorders associated with retinal detachment, angioid streaks, retinitis pigmentosa, congenital cataract or lens subluxation are covered elsewhere in this book.

ALBINISM

Albinism is characterised by reduced pigmentation of the eyes due to absence or abnormality of the tyrosinase enzyme responsible for converting tyrosine to melanin. It is termed

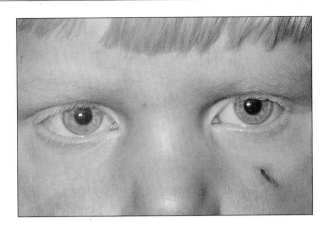

Figure 15.15
Oculocutaneous albinism

ocular albinism when the eyes alone are affected and *oculocutaneous* if skin involvement is present (Fig. 15.15). Ocular albinism is inherited as an X-linked recessive trait whilst oculocutaneous albinism tends to be autosomal recessive. Ocular features include nystagmus, strabismus, iris transillumination and depigmented fundus. Patients have stable, moderately reduced vision due to foveal hypoplasia and nystagmus.

GOUT

The hyperuricaemia that causes gout may be associated with band keratopathy, iritis, episcleritis and scleritis. Attacks of scleritis are the most important association and often accompany or precede joint involvement.

TAY–SACH'S DISEASE

Tay–Sach's disease is one of the autosomal recessively inherited gangliosidoses which usually affects Ashkenazi Jews. Patients present within the first year of life with progressive neurological disease. The classic ophthalmic finding is of a cherry-red spot at the macula.

WILSON'S DISEASE

Wilson's disease is characterised by widespread tissue deposition of copper in association with a deficiency of alpha-2-globulin. Clinically it may present with neurological or hepatic disease.

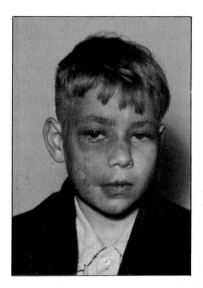

Figure 15.16
Facial angioma ('port-wine stain')

Ocular features include the deposition of copper in the deep layers of the peripheral cornea (Kayser–Fleischer ring), and the crystalline lens (sunflower cataract).

PHACOMATOSES

The phacomatoses are a group of disorders in which hamartomas are spread throughout the central nervous system, retina and skin.

- **von Hippel-Lindau syndrome**. This is an autosomal dominantly inherited condition characterised by the development of retinal and cerebellar angiomas. Visual loss may occur when fluid leaking from the retinal lesion affects the macula. The angiomas may be treated with laser photocoagulation or cryotheraphy. Affected patients should have annual screening for the development of retinal and cerebellar angiomas, phaeochromocytoma and hypernephroma.

- **Neurofibromatosis**. Neurofibromatosis occurs in two forms. Type 1 (von Recklinghausen's disease) patients have café au lait spots, axillary freckling and skin neurofibromas. Ocular features include ptosis (from lid neurofibromas), proptosis, glaucoma, iris (Lisch) nodules, retinal astrocytomas and optic nerve gliomas. Patients with type 2 (central) neurofibromatosis develop bilateral acoustic neuromas and, occasionally, cataract.

- **Tuberose sclerosis**. This rare disease presents with adenoma sebaceum (small red nodules on the cheeks), epilepsy and mental retardation. Patients may develop astrocytic hamartomas of the retina.

- **Sturge–Weber syndrome**. This is an extensive unilateral port-wine naevus in the distribution of the first and second divisions of the Vth cranial nerve, in association with ipsilateral haemangiomas of the meninges and choroid and unilateral congenital glaucoma (Fig. 15.16).

Index